Orthodontics in 2025: Evidence Based Clinical Practice

Azhar ul Haque Sario

AF706129

Copyright

First Printing, 2025

Azhar.sario@hotmail.co.uk

ORCID: https://orcid.org/0009-0004-8629-830X
Disclaimer: This book is free from AI use. The cover was designed in Canva.

Disclaimer: The author of this work is not affiliated, associated, authorized, endorsed by, or in any way officially connected with the University of Pennsylvania, New York University (NYU), Saint Louis University (SLU), Jefferson Health, Columbia University, University of Illinois Chicago (UIC), the University of Michigan, Seton Hill University, or the University of the Pacific. All institutional and company names are used for identification and descriptive purposes only, under the principle of nominative fair use. This is an independently produced publication.

Contents

Part I: Foundational Paradigms in Modern Orthodontics

The New Patient Examination: Integrating Digital Diagnostics and Systemic Health

Your Smile Is a Story. What Is It Saying?

Look in the mirror. Past the reflection, past the familiar features, and focus on your smile. We've been taught to see it as a simple arrangement of teeth—straight or crooked, white or not. But what if your smile is telling a much deeper story? What if it's the cover of a book about your entire well-being, whispering secrets about how you breathe, how you sleep, and how you feel?

Welcome to the new frontier of orthodontics. The days of simply forcing teeth into a line are fading into the rearview mirror. Today's visionary orthodontists are less like tooth mechanics and more like facial architects. They understand that your mouth is not an island; it's the bustling capital city of your head and face, intricately connected to the highways of your airways and the very foundation of your jaw. This isn't just about straightening teeth; it's about building a healthier, more harmonious you.

Listening to the Foundation: The Secrets of Your Jaw

Before a single wire is placed, the examination begins with a gentle conversation—not with you, but with your jaw joints. Tucked just in front of your ears, the temporomandibular joints (TMJs) are the unsung heroes of your face, the powerful hinges that let you laugh, eat, and express every emotion.

But sometimes, these hardworking joints carry hidden burdens. An orthodontist listens for their story. Do they speak with a subtle click or a quiet pop? Is there a tenderness that hints at stress or strain? Does your jaw swing on a graceful, silent arc, or does it wander, deviating from its path as if searching for a more comfortable home?

These aren't minor quirks; they are vital clues. An unstable foundation can compromise the entire structure. That's why premier training programs dedicate so much time to this art of listening, ensuring that creating a beautiful smile doesn't come at the cost of your jaw's comfort and health. It's about ensuring the masterpiece has a foundation that will last a lifetime.

The Breath of Life: The Unseen Sculptor

Now, take a breath. Did you breathe through your nose or your mouth? This simple, unconscious act is one of the most powerful forces shaping your face. Breathing is the unseen sculptor, and how you do it matters immensely.

Ideally, we are nasal breathers. The nose is a miraculous filter, warming and purifying the air while promoting the balanced, forward growth of our facial structures. But when nasal passages are blocked—perhaps by oversized tonsils or chronic allergies—the body finds a workaround: mouth breathing.

An observant orthodontist becomes a detective, spotting the tell-tale signs. The parted lips at rest, the tell-tale shadows under the eyes, the long, narrow face—these are clues that the body is struggling for air. This can lead to a cascade of issues, from inflamed gums to a far more serious condition known as sleep-disordered breathing (SDB). SDB can disrupt sleep, strain the heart, and in children, affect everything from growth to their ability to focus in school.

While an orthodontist doesn't treat SDB, they are often the first line of defense, the vigilant professional who can spot the warning signs and guide you to the right specialists. It's a profound responsibility that looks beyond the mouth and into the very essence of your health.

The Artistry of the Face: Beyond a Perfect Bite

For decades, the ultimate prize in orthodontics was the "perfect bite." While essential, it's like having a perfectly engineered engine in a car with no regard for the car's design. Today, the focus has zoomed out to encompass the entire face. The real goal is harmony.

A modern orthodontist is also an artist. They study the landscape of your face—its unique proportions, its symmetry, the elegant curve of your chin, and the way your lips meet when you smile. Does the arc of your upper teeth follow the gentle curve of your lower lip? This is the "smile arc," a hallmark of a truly natural and radiant smile.

Your treatment is a collaboration, a process guided by your desires for a smile that doesn't just look straight, but looks like yours. It's a smile that fits the canvas of your face, creating a balanced, captivating profile that feels as good as it looks.

The Masterpiece of You

Putting it all together is the philosophy of treating the "whole patient." It's the understanding that the jaw, the airway, the teeth, and the face are not separate puzzles but a single, interconnected masterpiece. It's recognizing that the child with allergies might need more than just braces, and the adult who grinds their teeth needs a plan that protects their jaw joints.

The orthodontist of today has evolved. They are your health detective, your facial architect, and your personal artist. They are trained to see the whole story, to understand the deep connections between a beautiful smile and a vibrant life.

So the next time you look in the mirror, see more than just your teeth. See the intricate, beautiful, and complex story of you. And know that modern orthodontic care is dedicated to making every chapter a healthy and happy one.

For generations, the art of orthodontics was a bit like trying to understand a magnificent cathedral by studying only its blueprint and a few flat photographs. Clinicians, for all their skill, were working in a world of shadows and echoes. They peered at ghostly two-dimensional X-rays, trying to decipher the intricate, three-dimensional truth of a human face. They worked with heavy plaster models—brittle, chalky ghosts of a patient's smile. It was a craft of immense dedication, but one defined by its limits, by what couldn't be seen.

Then, light broke through the flatland. The arrival of three-dimensional imaging wasn't just another step forward; it was like discovering a whole new dimension of sight. This shift gave birth to a modern masterpiece of diagnostics: the "digital patient," a virtual, living sculpture built not from clay or plaster, but from pure, unadulterated data.

Peering Beneath the Surface: The Gift of X-Ray Vision

At the heart of this revolution is a technology that sounds like something from a sci-fi novel: Cone Beam Computed Tomography (CBCT). Think of it as giving an orthodontist a form of superpower. Where a traditional X-ray is a flat shadow puppet, a CBCT scan is a fully explorable, holographic map of the head. It peels back the skin, muscle, and gums to reveal the hidden architecture beneath—the elegant sweep of the jawbone, the precise position of every tooth root, the delicate pathways of nerves.

Suddenly, mysteries that once required educated guesswork are laid bare. That stubborn canine tooth that refuses to emerge? CBCT reveals its exact location, its angle, its relationship with its neighbors, transforming a high-stakes surgical puzzle into a clear and predictable path. For patients with complex facial asymmetries or those needing jaw surgery, this technology is nothing short of transformative. Surgeons and orthodontists can now walk through a complex procedure virtually, planning every minute adjustment on a digital replica before ever making an incision, ensuring the final result is not just functional, but harmonious.

Of course, this power comes with a profound responsibility—the use of radiation. This is where the guiding principle of "As Low As Reasonably Achievable" (ALARA) becomes paramount. It's a promise to the patient: to use the absolute minimum exposure necessary to get the vital information needed. Modern machines are masters of this, targeting only the specific area of interest, like a spotlight in a dark room. In the right hands, for the right case, the clarity it provides is a beacon of safety and predictability that far outshines the minimal, managed risk.

The Magic Wand of First Impressions

If CBCT reveals the hidden foundation, the intraoral scanner (IOS) has revolutionized how we see the visible smile. For nearly a century, getting a model of a patient's teeth was a primitive ritual. It involved filling the mouth with a cold, goopy, gag-inducing paste, an ordeal patients endured with clenched hands and watering eyes. The resulting plaster model was a fragile, imperfect relic.

Today, that entire messy chapter is being replaced by the sweep of a sleek digital wand. An intraoral scanner glides effortlessly over the teeth, using light to "paint" a perfect, high-definition digital portrait of every groove and contour in seconds. The experience for the patient is night-and-day: it's faster, cleaner, and profoundly more comfortable. The resulting digital file is flawless, immune to the warping or breaking that plagued its plaster ancestor.

But as of 2025, these wands do more than just see the surface. They now see into it. Using technologies like near-infrared light (NIRI), a scanner can illuminate the earliest signs of a cavity, often long before it's visible to the naked eye. They can become meticulous timekeepers, comparing scans over months or years to precisely measure the microscopic loss from tooth grinding. The IOS is no longer just a replacement for goop; it's a dynamic guardian of oral health.

The Grand Unification: Sculpting the Digital You

Herein lies the true magic. We have the skeleton from CBCT, the exquisite detail of the teeth from the IOS, and a third piece of the puzzle: a 3D facial scan that captures the soft, living landscape of the face. Each tells a vital part of the story, but each is incomplete on its own.

The real innovation is weaving these separate threads of data into a single, breathtaking tapestry. Sophisticated software now acts as a master weaver, intelligently fusing these datasets together. The bone, the teeth, and the face are layered and locked into their perfect anatomical relationship, creating a single, holistic model—a "Digital You."

This is the ultimate answer to the limitations of the past. It's a virtual replica of the patient, so complete and accurate that it becomes the foundational clay for the orthodontist's artistry. It's not just a static image; it's a dynamic sandbox. Here, the orthodontist becomes an architect of the future smile. They can gently move a digital tooth into its ideal home and watch how the change might affect the lip posture. They can simulate an entire 18-month treatment plan, exploring different paths and visualizing the final masterpiece before the journey even begins.

This digital twin becomes a bridge of understanding between doctor and patient. Instead of pointing at a confusing X-ray, an orthodontist can now sit with a patient, rotate their "Digital You" on a screen, and say, "This is where we are, and this is the beautiful, healthy smile we can create together." It replaces apprehension with collaboration, confusion with clarity.

While the path to this digital future has its hurdles—the cost of entry, the steep learning curve, the challenge of managing vast amounts of data—they are the price of admission to this new world. Looking ahead, the horizon is electric with possibility. Artificial intelligence is beginning to act as a wise collaborator, analyzing these digital twins to spot subtle issues and suggest optimal strategies. The dream of a truly bespoke smile, where every bracket, every aligner, every movement is custom-designed based on a patient's unique digital blueprint, is no longer a dream. It's the new reality. We have moved from tracing shadows on a cave wall to sculpting with light itself.

The Ghost in the Machine: How AI is Becoming the Orthodontist's New Superpower

For generations, the art of orthodontics lived in the quiet hum of a light-box and the delicate dance of a clinician's hand. It was a world of tracing paper, sharpened pencils, and an almost intuitive ability to see through the flat, grayscale world of an X-ray to the complex, three-dimensional truth of a patient's smile. Every angle, every millimeter was a judgment call, a testament to years of training where the orthodontist's eye was the ultimate diagnostic tool. This was a craft of immense skill, but also one shadowed by the quiet ghost of human variability—the subtle tremor of a hand, the slight difference in perspective from one expert to the next.

Now, a new partner has entered the room, not with a pencil, but with the silent, processing power of a billion calculations a second. Artificial Intelligence is stepping out of the realm of science fiction and into the heart of the orthodontic practice, and it's not just changing the tools of the trade; it's transforming the very nature of diagnosis itself.

From Hand-Drawn Maps to Digital GPS

Think of the old way, the manual cephalometric analysis, as navigating a dense forest with a hand-drawn map. It was reliable, born of experience, but slow and subject to the mapmaker's interpretation. A clinician would spend painstaking minutes, hunched over a headfilm, marking landmarks like the "sella" or the "nasion"—key points on the skull that act as the stars by which they navigate a treatment plan. It was a ritual of precision, but one that could now be accomplished in the time it takes to draw a single breath.

AI has become the GPS. Fed on a diet of tens of thousands of expertly analyzed images, these sophisticated algorithms have learned to see the invisible architecture of the human face with breathtaking speed and consistency. They don't get tired. They don't have an off day. They can pinpoint those crucial anatomical landmarks with an accuracy that hovers around 90%, effectively banishing the ghost of inter-operator variability. The result is a diagnostic foundation that is standardized, objective, and incredibly fast, freeing the orthodontist from the meticulous labor of map-making to focus on the journey ahead.

Seeing in Three Dimensions: The Unseen World Revealed

But AI's true magic isn't just about doing the old things faster. It's about seeing things that were once impossible to see. With the advent of Cone Beam Computed Tomography (CBCT), orthodontists were handed a treasure trove of data—a complete 3D digital model of their patient. It was like going from a single photograph to a fully explorable, holographic replica of the skull, teeth, and soft tissues. The problem? It was too much information, a dazzling universe of data that could overwhelm the human eye.

Here, AI acts as a tireless deep-sea explorer, plunging into the depths of this data to find what might otherwise be missed. It can spot the faintest shadows of root resorption, identify the precise location of an impacted tooth hiding deep within the jaw, or even measure the airway to flag potential breathing problems that could impact a child's health and development. It's a second set of eyes, unburdened by fatigue, that can detect subtle patterns across millions of data points. This doesn't just enhance diagnosis; it elevates it, transforming it from an act of interpretation to one of profound discovery.

The Human Touch: Why the Artist is More Important Than Ever

It's tempting to view this as the dawn of the robot orthodontist, but that would be missing the most beautiful part of the story. AI, for all its power, is still a tool. And like any tool, it has its limits. It is only as wise as the data it was trained on, and recent studies show it can still be flummoxed by the subtle nuances of reality—like the precise tilt of an incisor that a human expert can intuitively understand.

This is where the orthodontist's role is not diminished but brilliantly redefined. The primary clinical skill is no longer just about deciphering shadows on a film. It's about becoming a masterful interpreter of a powerful algorithm. It's knowing when to trust the machine's incredible output and when to challenge it, guided by the one thing the AI will never have: human experience.

The modern orthodontist stands at the confluence of two worlds. In one hand, they hold a universe of objective, quantifiable data from the AI—a perfect, digital blueprint of the patient's anatomy. But in the other, they hold the unquantifiable, exquisitely human factors: the patient's dreams for their smile, their anxieties about treatment, their lifestyle, and their unique biology.

The true art of diagnosis in this new era is the synthesis of these two worlds. It is the ability to look at the flawless data and then turn to the person in the chair, blending the science of the algorithm with the empathy of the human heart. It's using the machine's precision to build the plan, but using human wisdom to make it a plan that fits a life.

The future is a duet. AI will do the heavy lifting, the complex calculations, and the tireless searching. But the orthodontist will provide the soul. This collaborative dance between human and machine promises a future where every patient's journey to a new smile is more precise, more insightful, and more profoundly human than ever before.

The Conductor of the Smile

Forget everything you thought you knew about the orthodontist. Banish the image of a technician tightening wires in a sterile room, focused only on the clockwork of teeth. Today, that picture is as outdated as a flip phone. Step instead into the grand concert hall of your own body, and see the orthodontist for who they truly are: a conductor.

Your body is a symphony, a breathtakingly complex orchestra where every system, every organ, every cell plays its part. Your heartbeat provides the steady percussion, your lungs the sweeping woodwinds, your nervous system the intricate strings. And the mouth? The mouth is the stage itself, the resonant chamber through which so much of this music is expressed. It's where the first notes of trouble often sound, long before the rest of the orchestra falls into discord.

The modern orthodontist is trained to listen to this music with a uniquely attuned ear. They are no longer just concerned with the alignment of the ivories; they are listening for the harmony of your entire being.

Think of a patient who snores, whose sleep is a nightly battle for breath. This isn't just a noisy nuisance; it's a stutter in the orchestra's rhythm, a sign that the airway—the vital wind section—is being muffled. A traditional view might see only a narrow jaw. The modern orthodontist sees a potential link to sleep apnea and its cascade of serious health issues, from heart strain to chronic fatigue. They don't just act alone; they pick up their baton and co-conduct a masterpiece of care with sleep doctors and ear, nose, and throat specialists, perhaps introducing a custom oral appliance that silently, elegantly, reopens the airway and lets the music of healthy breathing play on through the night.

Consider the foundation of the smile: the delicate, vital gums and bone that anchor each tooth. An orthodontist who simply applies braces without examining this foundation is like a conductor ignoring a crack in the stage floor. The pressure of moving teeth can turn a minor gum issue into a full-blown crisis of inflammation and bone loss. That is why the partnership with a periodontist (a gum specialist) is now a sacred pact. It's a powerful duet, ensuring the stage is strong and healthy before the dance of realignment even begins. Esteemed schools like Penn Dental Medicine are built on this philosophy, teaching that a beautiful smile on an unhealthy foundation is a hollow victory.

Nowhere is this collaborative spirit more profound than in the lives of children born with craniofacial differences like a cleft lip or palate. Here, the orthodontist is a first-chair musician in a vast, lifelong symphony of healing. From infancy through adulthood, they work in seamless harmony with plastic surgeons, speech pathologists, and geneticists. They are the architects of the jaw, the guides of growth, the artists who ensure that a child's smile is not a source of struggle, but a triumphant crescendo in their life's unique composition.

The truth is, the mouth is a living storybook of our systemic health. The pale hue of the gums might speak of anemia. A persistently dry mouth could be a whisper of an autoimmune condition. The very landscape of the tongue can betray a nutritional deficiency. The orthodontist, with their focused view, is often the first to read these subtle sentences. They have become essential scouts on the frontier of our well-being, raising a flag that guides a patient toward the right medical expert, sometimes changing—or even saving—a life through early detection.

So, the next time you think of an orthodontic exam, picture more than just molds and X-rays. See it as a comprehensive wellness check-in, a moment where a dedicated professional leans in to listen to your body's symphony. They are listening for the rhythm of your sleep, the health of your core, and the silent signals your body is sending.

This is the art and soul of modern orthodontics. It's a commitment that goes far beyond the mechanics of a smile to embrace the health of a whole person. It is a more challenging, more profound, and infinitely more rewarding score to play. The result isn't just straight teeth; it's a body and a life brought into greater harmony. And that is a beautiful music, indeed.

The Biological Basis of Tooth Movement: From Cellular Mechanics to Epigenetic Influences

The Secret Life of a Tooth: A Story of Push, Pull, and Remaking Yourself

Your teeth aren't just pegs hammered into your jaw. Forget that image entirely. Instead, picture each tooth as a dancer, poised and ready, suspended in a delicate, living sling. This remarkable partner is the periodontal ligament, or PDL, a tissue so full of life it practically hums. It's not just a rope; it's a bustling communication hub, a vibrant network of feeling, blood flow, and raw potential that connects your tooth to the bone that holds it. And it's within this whispered conversation between tooth, ligament, and bone that the magic of orthodontics truly happens.

When an orthodontist gently nudges a tooth, they aren't just shoving it. They are initiating a profound dialogue. The force is a message, sent through the PDL, that whispers to the surrounding bone: "We need to move." This signal sparks a biological ballet known as the pressure-tension theory, a story of yielding and rebuilding that reshapes your smile from the inside out.

The Give: A Courteous Retreat

Imagine the tooth beginning its slow journey. On the side it's moving toward, the PDL feels a gentle squeeze. This is the "pressure side." It's not a painful crush, but a persistent, steady compression. The tiny blood vessels within the ligament narrow, and the area becomes a flurry of controlled activity. Think of it as the body politely asking the bone to step aside.

This request summons a team of incredible artist-cells called osteoclasts. They are not demolition crews, but masterful sculptors. Their job is to deconstruct, to dissolve the bone crystal by crystal, creating the precise space needed for the tooth's new home. They are the masters of the give, clearing a path not with brute force, but with intricate biological grace. Without their work, the tooth would be stuck, its journey halted before it could even begin.

The Take: Weaving a New Anchor

But for every give, there must be a take. As the tooth glides into its newly created space, the PDL on the opposite side stretches, like a line pulled taut. This is the "tension side," and here, the story is one of creation. The stretched fibers and healthy, flowing blood supply send out a different kind of signal—a call to build.

Answering this call are the osteoblasts, the architects of bone. Where the osteoclasts carved away, the osteoblasts arrive to weave anew. They spin out a fresh, pliable matrix called osteoid, which becomes the foundation for new bone. They are the keepers of integrity, ensuring that as the tooth moves, it is never left unsupported. They fill in the space behind, anchoring the tooth securely in its ever-changing position, a testament to the body's refusal to leave a job half-done.

The Rhythm of the Dance

This synchronized performance—the deconstruction on one side and the reconstruction on the other—is the very soul of orthodontic movement. It's a continuous, flowing rhythm of bone resorption and formation, a dance between yielding and becoming. This is why the force applied by an orthodontist must be so specific.

Think of it like training a delicate plant to grow along a trellis. Too little pressure, and the plant ignores you. The message is lost, the dance never begins. But too much force is a shock to the system. It can strangle the vital blood supply to the PDL, causing a kind of cellular burnout where movement just stops. This can lead to discomfort and even damage the tooth's root or the surrounding bone.

The duration matters, too. The cellular dancers need a consistent rhythm. An intermittent force is like a conductor who keeps stopping and starting the music; the osteoclasts and osteoblasts become confused, and the beautiful remodeling process falters. This is why wearing your aligners or appliance as prescribed is so critical—it maintains the constant, gentle persuasion needed for the bone to reshape itself willingly.

Ultimately, moving a tooth is a profound collaboration with your own body. It's a process built on respect for the intricate, living systems that govern our biology. It's not about forcing change, but about inviting it. By applying a precise and gentle nudge, orthodontics taps into this incredible, innate intelligence—this beautiful, biological dance—to guide your smile toward a new horizon.

The Secret Life of Your Teeth: The Unsung Hero of a Perfect Smile

We all marvel at the magic of orthodontics—the slow, steady journey from a crowded smile to a perfectly aligned set of pearly whites. It feels like a work of art, and it is. But behind every beautiful smile is a hidden force, a silent hero working tirelessly in the background. This hero isn't the shiny braces or the clear aligners; it's a concept called anchorage.

Think of it this way: imagine you're on a small raft and you need to pull a friend's raft closer to you. When you pull on their rope, what happens? You both drift towards each other. Neither of you has a stable anchor. Now, imagine you're standing firmly on a pier. When you pull the rope, only your friend's raft moves. You are the anchor—the unmoving, reliable base.

In the world of your mouth, orthodontics is a constant, gentle tug-of-war. To move one tooth, we must have an unmoving pier to pull from. That pier is anchorage. It's the art of keeping some teeth stock-still so that others can glide gracefully into their new homes. This idea, which truly came to life in the mid-20th century, is the invisible foundation upon which your entire treatment is built.

A Tug-of-War Governed by Nature's Law

At the heart of this challenge is a law you learned in high school science class: Newton's Third Law. For every action, there is an equal and opposite reaction. When your orthodontist applies a force to guide a wayward tooth (the "active" tooth), that force doesn't just disappear. It bounces back, pushing against the teeth used for stability (the "anchor" teeth).

If the anchor teeth give in to this reactive push and start drifting themselves, we call it "anchorage loss." It's like the pier starting to crumble and slide into the water. This can compromise the whole plan, turning a precisely calculated treatment into a frustrating game of dental whack-a-mole.

The Jawbone's Construction Crew: A Biological Ballet

But how does a tooth actually move? It's not just brute force. It's a breathtakingly intricate biological ballet happening deep within your jawbone. Your tooth isn't fused directly to the bone; it's nestled in a socket, cushioned by a remarkable living tissue called the periodontal ligament, or PDL. Think of the PDL as a tiny, intelligent trampoline that holds your tooth in place.

When a gentle, continuous pressure is applied to a tooth, this trampoline gets squished on one side and stretched on the other. This change in pressure is a signal, a call to action for a specialized crew of cells living in the surrounding bone.

On the side where the PDL is compressed, a "demolition crew" of cells called osteoclasts arrives. Their mission? To dissolve tiny bits of bone, clearing a path for the tooth to move. It's a slow, meticulous excavation.

Meanwhile, on the tension side where the PDL is stretched, a "construction crew" of osteoblasts gets to work. These master builders lay down new bone, filling in the space the tooth just left. This constant, coordinated process of bone removal and creation is called bone remodeling. It's the living, breathing engine that allows your orthodontist to sculpt your smile.

The Wisdom of the Roots: Nature's Anchors

So, what makes a tooth a sturdy pier rather than a wobbly raft? The secret lies beneath the gum line: the root surface area.

A big, old oak tree with a deep, sprawling root system is nearly impossible to move. A small sapling with a single, shallow root? Much easier. It's the same in your mouth. Your mighty molars, with their large, multiple roots, are like the oak trees of your jaw. They have a massive surface area gripping the bone, making them naturally resistant to movement. Your incisors and premolars, with their smaller, single roots, are more like the saplings.

This is why your back teeth have traditionally been the anchors of choice. They are the heavyweight champions, capable of resisting the reactive forces of the orthodontic tug-of-war.

The Art of the Gentle Nudge

This biological reality gives rise to the "differential force theory." It's a strategy of finesse over force. By applying a light, gentle nudge to the teeth we want to move, we can get them to glide along without waking the sleeping giants—the anchor molars. The force is just enough to signal the demolition and construction crews to get to work on the smaller tooth, but not strong enough to budge the larger, more stubborn anchor.

But even with this clever approach, relying on other teeth for anchorage is never a sure bet. The body is a dynamic system. Over time, even the strongest molar might shift just a little, a tiny concession in the tug-of-war. This is the constant challenge that keeps orthodontists on their toes.

When Anchors Need Superpowers: Headgear and a Modern Marvel

For decades, when a case required truly immovable anchorage, orthodontists looked outside the mouth. The solution was headgear, an appliance that transferred the reactive forces to the back of the head or neck. By anchoring to the skull, headgear provided a truly stable point, allowing for major tooth movements that were impossible with teeth alone. While incredibly effective, headgear's reliance on patient cooperation and its visible nature made it a less-than-popular option.

Then came a revolution. A game-changer that has transformed the field: Temporary Anchorage Devices (TADs).

TADs are tiny, biocompatible screws, no bigger than an earring stud, that are placed directly into the jawbone. Their genius is in their simplicity. Instead of using a tooth (which is designed to move), a TAD uses the bone itself as the anchor. It's like drilling a permanent hook into a concrete wall. When you pull on that hook, the wall doesn't move.

This "skeletal anchorage" is virtually absolute. The TAD becomes one with the bone, providing an unyielding point of stability. With TADs, orthodontists can now perform feats that once seemed like science fiction:

Intruding teeth: Pushing them back up into the bone to correct a gummy smile.

Distalizing molars: Moving an entire line of teeth backward to create space.

Closing large gaps without the front teeth drifting forward.

TADs give orthodontists unparalleled control, allowing them to focus all the force precisely where it's needed, eliminating the worry of anchorage loss. They are the silent, invisible superheroes that make complex treatments simpler, faster, and more predictable.

The Foundation of Your Future Smile

From the cellular construction crews to the physics of force, anchorage is the unseen science and unsung hero behind your orthodontic journey. It is the deep understanding of biology that allows your orthodontist to be not just a doctor, but an artist—sculpting with bone, guiding with gentle force, and building a foundation for a beautiful, healthy smile that will last a lifetime. The next time you see someone with braces, remember the quiet, powerful ballet happening just beneath the surface, a testament to the incredible partnership between human ingenuity and the wisdom of the body.

The Unwritten Story of Your Face: How Life Shapes the Way We Look

We used to think the story of our face was written in stone, etched into the unchangeable code of our DNA. We looked at our parents, saw our future jawline, the set of our teeth, and simply accepted it as destiny. But 2025 has torn that book from our hands and revealed a truth that is both simpler and far more profound: our own lives are the ghostwriters of our biology.

This revolution is called epigenetics, and it's about the remarkable power of our experiences to conduct the orchestra of our genes. Imagine your DNA isn't a rigid blueprint, but a vast musical score. Epigenetics is the conductor, choosing which instruments to bring to the forefront and which to quiet, all based on the environment you live in, the food you eat, and even the way you breathe. This isn't about changing the notes themselves, but about interpreting the music in a way that creates a unique and personal symphony. In the world of orthodontics, this is more than a new chapter; it's a whole new story, one where the shape of our face is not just inherited, but earned.

The Silent Sculptor in Your Mouth

If you want to witness this epic story unfold, look no further than the unsung hero—or potential villain—of our facial development: the tongue. It's a powerhouse of a muscle, a tireless sculptor that, when resting correctly, presses gently against the roof of our mouth. This subtle, constant pressure is the secret architect of a wide, healthy upper jaw, creating the perfect, spacious landscape for our teeth to settle into. It's nature's own palate expander, working silently, day and night.

But what happens when a child can't breathe through their nose? An allergy, a cold, or swollen adenoids can force them to become a "mouth breather." In this seemingly minor shift, the entire architectural plan changes. The tongue, no longer able to rest in its rightful place, drops to the floor of the mouth to clear a path for air. The sculptor abandons its post.

Without that gentle, expansive force, the upper jaw, the maxilla, follows a different path. It grows narrow and high, like a Gothic arch instead of a Roman one. The consequence is a story told in dental offices every day: crowded, crooked teeth, a recessed chin, and a cascade of other issues. This isn't bad genetic luck. It's a direct, physical outcome of a functional habit—a powerful testament to how the way we use our bodies fundamentally shapes our form.

A Symphony of Whispers

The tongue's tale is just one verse in a much larger epic. Our development is a symphony of environmental whispers, each one influencing the genetic melody.

Think about our modern diet. Our ancestors chewed tough, fibrous foods, giving their jaws a daily workout that stimulated strong, robust bone growth. Today, our world is one of smoothies, processed grains, and soft textures. Our jaws, in a sense, have become couch potatoes. Without the vigorous stimulation of chewing, the genetic potential for a broad, powerful jaw can remain dormant, leading to crowding and misalignment even in those with "perfect" genes.

This story begins even before birth. A mother's diet, her stress levels, the very air she breathes—these all send epigenetic signals to her developing child. A deficiency in something as simple as folic acid can influence how the genes responsible for facial fusion are expressed. It's not that the gene is "bad," but that the environment didn't provide the right cues at the right time.

Even the first act of life, nursing, plays a part. The intricate dance of muscles required for breastfeeding is a perfect workout for a developing infant's jaw and promotes the habit of nasal breathing. In contrast, certain bottle nipples or extended pacifier use can retrain these muscles in less optimal ways, subtly altering the course of facial growth. From the womb to the dinner table, our lives are in constant dialogue with our DNA.

The Tiny Conductors and the Power to Retrain

Scientists, peering deeper into this molecular world, have discovered the tiny conductors of this symphony:

microRNAs. These aren't genes themselves, but microscopic maestros that can silence or amplify genetic messages. They are the ones who tell a developing tooth when to grow, when to stop, and where to go.

We are now finding that issues like missing teeth (tooth agenesis) aren't always a simple case of a missing gene, but may be a problem of regulation—a microRNA conductor that is out of tune. This discovery is a game-changer. Imagine a future where we don't just mechanically move teeth after they've grown in crookedly, but where we can target these tiny regulators to guide development from the very beginning, correcting potential anomalies at a molecular level.

This brings us to the most empowering part of this new chapter: myofunctional therapy. If bad habits can steer growth off course, then good habits can guide it back. Myofunctional therapy is essentially physical therapy for the face, tongue, and lips. It's a series of simple, targeted exercises that retrain the body for optimal function. It teaches a mouth-breathing child how to breathe through their nose, how to seal their lips, and, most importantly, how to restore their tongue to its rightful throne against the palate.

By correcting the root cause of the dysfunction, myofunctional therapy doesn't just treat the symptoms; it rebuilds the foundation. It can:

Liberate Jaw Growth: By placing the tongue back in its role as a natural palate expander, it encourages the jaws to grow to their full, beautiful potential.

Open Airways: Establishing nasal breathing is life-changing, improving sleep, reducing the risk of sleep apnea, and even boosting cognitive function.

Create Lasting Harmony: When orthodontics are needed, this therapy helps ensure the results are stable, preventing relapse by correcting the very muscle patterns that caused the problem in the first place.

The Dawn of the Growth Guide

This epigenetic understanding is shifting the very soul of orthodontics. The orthodontist is no longer just a mechanic for the mouth, reacting to problems after they arise. They are becoming proactive guides of growth, preventative architects of the face.

The future of a healthy smile isn't about waiting for crooked teeth to appear and then bracing them into submission. It's about looking at a child and seeing not a fixed destiny, but a dynamic process. It's about spotting the subtle signs of improper function early on and intervening with gentle, guiding forces. It's a future that promises less invasive treatments, more stable results, and a deeper appreciation for the intricate, beautiful dance between our lives and our biology. We are finally learning that the story of our face is not one that is written for us, but one that we have the power to help write ourselves.

The Smile Architect and the Living Blueprint: A Deeper Look at Moving Mountains (and Teeth)

Orthodontic treatment is a kind of magic, isn't it? It's the quiet, patient art of convincing teeth to journey to new homes, transforming not just a smile, but the very landscape of a person's oral health. But this is no simple sleight of hand. We are not working with inert blocks of enamel, but with a living, breathing system—a dynamic ecosystem of bone, ligaments, and nerves. Every gentle nudge from a wire, every subtle pressure from an aligner, is a conversation with the body.

And like any profound conversation, it carries inherent risks. When we ask the body to remodel itself, we are initiating a powerful biological cascade. These are the "iatrogenic" risks—the body's own protests and adaptations to the forces we apply. Two of these conversations demand our utmost respect and attention: the silent shortening of a tooth's anchor, known as root resorption, and the delicate dance of maintaining healthy gums, the very foundation of it all. To be a true architect of smiles is to first be a student of this profound biological dialogue, ensuring our work is not just effective, but deeply and fundamentally safe.

The Anchor's Slow Fade: Understanding the Body's Price for Movement

Picture a tooth's root not just as a peg, but as the deep, vital anchor of a mighty ship, holding it steady against the tides. External apical root resorption (EARR) is the gradual, often invisible, shortening of this anchor. A minuscule amount is a common and harmless whisper from the body, but when the whisper becomes a shout, it can compromise the tooth's future, leaving it less stable in the jaw. It's like discovering the foundation of your home has been quietly eroding for years—the structure might still be standing, but its resilience is in question.

What causes this silent fading? The story is written in the space between tooth and bone, in a thin, vital tissue called the periodontal ligament (PDL). When we apply orthodontic force, we squeeze this ligament. If the pressure is too strong or relentless, it's like stepping on a garden hose—the life-giving blood supply is temporarily cut off.

The cells in this compressed zone, starved of oxygen, can perish, creating a small, sterile wound.

Our body, the ultimate first responder, senses this damage and dispatches a specialized cleanup crew. These cells, known as osteoclasts and cementoclasts, are microscopic miracle workers, designed to dissolve and remove damaged tissue. But sometimes, in their determined effort to clear away the wreckage, they become overzealous. They can't perfectly distinguish between the damaged tissue and the healthy surface of the tooth's root. In their mission to heal, they inadvertently begin to sand away the very anchor they are meant to protect. It's a biological paradox—a healing process that can cause unintended harm, a renovation crew that accidentally chips away at the cornerstone.

Tipping the Scales: Who Walks the Tightrope of Risk?

While this microscopic drama unfolds in every orthodontic patient, some are more likely to experience a significant fade in their tooth anchors. Understanding these risk factors is like knowing the weather before setting sail.

First, there is the nature of the force itself. Imagine trying to move a boulder. A series of gentle, rhythmic pushes is far less likely to cause damage than a single, violent shove. In the same way, heavy, unrelenting orthodontic forces are the primary culprits. The longer the treatment, the more time the "cleanup crew" has to get overzealous. Certain movements, like pushing a tooth down into the bone or applying significant twisting force to the root, are like asking the body to perform its most complex and risky maneuvers.

But the story isn't just about the orthodontist; it's also about the patient's unique biological blueprint. Our genes can write a predisposition for risk into our very cells. Some of us, due to variations in our inflammatory response genes, are simply programmed to react more aggressively to orthodontic pressure. Systemic health plays a role, too; conditions like thyroid dysfunction can change the body's internal chemistry, making it more susceptible. Even the shape of the tooth's root matters—slender, pointed, or already short roots are like anchors that were forged with less material to begin with. A history of dental trauma is like a pre-existing fracture in the foundation, a vulnerability waiting to be exposed.

We keep watch over this process with the careful eye of a cartographer, using X-rays to map the landscape of the roots before, during, and after the journey. These images are our windows into the silent, unseen world beneath the gums.

Guarding the Garden: Why Gum Health is Everything

The periodontium—the gums, ligament, and bone—is the living soil in which our teeth are planted. Its health is the absolute prerequisite for any orthodontic endeavor. Moving teeth is, in essence, an act of controlled gardening, and you can't transplant a prize rose into diseased soil.

In a healthy mouth, orthodontics can be a gift to the gums. Uncrowding teeth makes them easier to clean, starving the harmful bacteria that cause inflammation. Correcting a misaligned bite distributes chewing forces more equitably, preventing certain teeth from bearing an unjust burden.

But attempting to move a tooth in the presence of active gum disease is like trying to build a skyscraper during an earthquake. The existing inflammation is a raging fire, and orthodontic forces act as a powerful accelerant. Instead of predictable movement, you get a catastrophic acceleration of bone loss, potentially dooming the tooth.

This is why a meticulous periodontal exam isn't just a good idea; it's a sacred pact between the clinician and the patient. Before a single wire is placed, we must ensure the foundation is sound. For patients with a history of gum disease, this often means a beautiful collaboration with a periodontist, a specialist in the health of this vital "soil." They are the master gardeners who ensure the ground is stable and ready for change. Only then, hand-in-hand, can we begin the journey of moving the teeth. We also pay close attention to patients with naturally thin, delicate gums. For them, moving teeth can be like stretching a fine fabric too far, potentially leading to recession. In these cases, we might proactively reinforce the gums with a graft, ensuring the garden remains lush and healthy for years to come.

The Light at the End of the Tunnel: Innovations in Gentler Journeys

The quest to make orthodontics safer and more attuned to our biology is perpetual. We are constantly learning the body's language, and with that knowledge, developing more sophisticated tools.

One of the most exciting new dialects we're learning is "photobiomodulation" (PBM), or low-level light therapy. By bathing the tissues in specific wavelengths of low-power light, we can have a remarkable conversation with our cells. This light seems to soothe the body's inflammatory response, encouraging a more efficient and less aggressive healing process. Studies suggest that this gentle encouragement can not only speed up tooth movement but also significantly protect the roots from resorption. It's like whispering to the body's cleanup crew, "Easy does it. Be precise. Heal, don't harm."

This is the future: a deeper partnership with the body. A future where treatment is personalized not just to a patient's bite, but to their unique genetic and biological identity.

The Promise of a Smile, The Pledge of a Steward

In the end, creating a beautiful smile is a profound responsibility. It requires us to be more than technicians; it requires us to be stewards of a living system. We must honor the biological conversation, mitigating the risks of root resorption and periodontal stress with every decision we make. This deep respect for the body's intricate dance is what transforms orthodontics from a mechanical procedure into a true healing art. It is a commitment to not only deliver a stunning result but to safeguard the health and integrity of that smile for a lifetime.

Advanced Biomechanics and Personalized Treatment Mechanics

The Tooth's Stubborn Heart: A Secret Dance in the Jaw

Every tooth has a secret. Buried deep beneath the gum line, nestled in the quiet dark of the jawbone, lies its true center of being. We call it the Center of Resistance (CRes), but it's more soulful than that. Think of it as the tooth's stubborn, unshakeable heart. It's the point of perfect balance, the silent fulcrum around which its entire life pivots.

If you could somehow whisper a command directly to this heart, the tooth would perform the simplest of movements. It would glide, pure and true, in the direction of your suggestion. A clean, honest slide, with no drama, no spin, no rotation. It would be a ghost-like movement, a perfect translation.

But life, and orthodontics, are never that simple. We can't speak directly to the tooth's heart. It's hidden, protected within the bone. Our conversation must happen on the surface, at the crown, where a bracket is bonded like a handshake. And because we are talking to the hand, not the heart, the tooth doesn't just slide. It begins to dance.

The Whisper and the Pirouette: Force and the Moment

The orthodontist's tool is Force, but it isn't a shout. It's a whisper. A gentle, continuous suggestion delivered through the fine architecture of wires, springs, and aligners. This whisper has a direction and a strength, a carefully calibrated question posed to the tooth and its supporting bone. Too loud, and the tissues become bruised and battered. Too soft, and the whisper is lost, ignored. The orthodontist seeks the perfect tone—a force that coaxes the bone to remodel, to yield, to create a new path.

This whisper, applied at the crown, never quite aligns with the tooth's hidden heart. And this beautiful misalignment, this distance between the asking force and the core of being, creates a Moment. A Moment is the soul of the dance. It's the tendency to turn, to spin, to pirouette. It's the twist in the plot.

Imagine a figure skater. A push from the side (the force) sends them gliding across the ice. But a push on their outstretched arm (a force applied at a distance from their center) makes them spin. The further out the push, the more dramatic the spin. That spin is the Moment. In orthodontics, a force is almost never just a push; it is always an invitation to a dance, a combination of a glide and a spin. The orthodontist's true genius lies not in applying the force, but in choreographing the spin.

The Choreographer's Code: The Moment-to-Force (M/F) Ratio

This is where science becomes art. The secret to controlling the dance lies in a single, elegant formula: the Moment-to-Force (M/F) Ratio. This ratio is the choreographer's code. It's the precise instruction that dictates the nature of every single step. By mastering this ratio, the orthodontist can command a full repertoire of movements, from a slight lean to a full-body glide, transforming a crooked smile into a masterpiece of living architecture.

Here is the choreography, decoded:

The Awkward Stumble (Low M/F Ratio): When the force is strong and the rotational moment is weak, the tooth performs an "uncontrolled tip." The crown, eager and impulsive, rushes forward in the direction of the force, while the root, its anchor, gets left behind, sometimes even swinging in the opposite direction. It's like a dancer stumbling forward, their head leading far ahead of their feet. It's a quick, easy move, sometimes useful for making a fast change, but lacks grace and stability if left unmanaged.

The Graceful Bow (Moderate M/F Ratio): With a more balanced M/F ratio, we get a "controlled tip." Here, the choreographer adds just enough spin to the push to tell the root, "Stay put." Imagine a dancer planting one foot firmly while their upper body bows elegantly. The crown tips into its new place, closing a gap or finding its alignment, while the root remains a stable, dignified anchor. This is a move of poise and intention.

The Perfect Glide (Specific M/F Ratio $\approx$ 10:1): This is the pas de deux, the flawless foxtrot of orthodontics. With an exquisitely precise M/F ratio, the orthodontist achieves bodily movement, or translation. The glide and the spin are in such perfect harmony that they cancel each other out, resulting in no rotation at all. The crown and the root move as one, a single unit gliding serenely through the bone, maintaining their perfect vertical posture. This is the masterful, challenging move required to shift entire sections of a smile without disturbing their orientation.

The Grounding Flourish (High M/F Ratio): Finally, we have torque, the dance of the root itself. Here, the rotational Moment is the star of the show, and the force is merely its quiet accompanist. By applying a sophisticated twist through the wire, the orthodontist can keep the crown almost perfectly still while speaking directly to the root, commanding it to move. This is the finishing flourish, the deep, grounding plié that settles the tooth into its final, perfect position within the bone. It's the unseen move that ensures not just a beautiful smile, but a stable, healthy, and lasting one.

The Artist-Engineer of the Human Smile

This is the world of the orthodontist. It is a world learned not from a simple manual, but through rigorous training in the biomechanical arts at institutions like SLU and Seton Hill. Here, they become more than doctors; they become artist-engineers.

They learn to read the secret language of each patient's biology. They diagnose not just crooked teeth, but the underlying forces and moments that created them. Then, with a deep understanding of this silent dance, they design a new choreography. They become interpreters of whispers and masters of the spin, constantly assessing, adjusting, and guiding. They are troubleshooting a complex biological system, turning a dance of disharmony into a symphony of alignment, health, and profound confidence.

The Smile's Secret Blueprint: How a Tiny Metal Square Changed Faces Forever

For most of modern history, creating a perfect smile was an act of pure artistry, a master craft practiced in the quiet hum of a dental office. An orthodontist wasn't just a doctor; they were a sculptor. Armed with pliers and a roll of wire, they would peer into a patient's mouth and begin a painstaking process of bending, twisting, and coaxing. Each tooth was a unique challenge, and every single wire was a hand-forged sculpture designed to move it. The process was long, arduous, and depended entirely on the almost magical dexterity of the clinician. A beautiful smile was possible, but the path to it was different every single time.

Then, in the 1970s, a revolutionary idea flipped that entire world on its head. It was a shift in thinking so profound it was almost philosophical. What if, instead of bending the wire to fit the teeth, we could tell the teeth where to go and let a simple, straight wire guide them home?

This was the birth of the Straight-Wire Appliance, and it wasn't just a new tool; it was a new way of seeing.

The Whisper of an Idea: Building the Map into the Bracket

The genius behind this leap belonged to Dr. Lawrence F. Andrews. He embarked on a quest, studying thousands of naturally perfect smiles, looking for a pattern, a universal truth. And he found it. He identified "The Six Keys to Normal Occlusion," a set of shared characteristics—the precise tilt, lean, and rotation—that defined a naturally ideal bite.

His insight was this: if we know the destination, why are we still drawing the map by hand for every journey?

Instead of the wire holding all the complex instructions, he imagined building those instructions directly into the brackets themselves. Each tiny metal square glued to a tooth would become a pre-programmed piece of hardware. The slot where the wire sits would be precisely angled and inclined, a tiny, built-in GPS whispering directions to the tooth. "Tilt forward just so," it would say. "Lean back a little. Rotate until you're perfectly aligned with your neighbors."

Suddenly, the orthodontist's job was no longer about being a master wire-bender. It was about becoming a master architect, meticulously placing these intelligent brackets to unlock the smile's hidden blueprint.

The Language of a Smile: Understanding the Prescription

At the core of this system is the "prescription"—a language of angles and dimensions baked into each bracket. It's the bracket's DNA, dictating how it will guide the tooth once a wire is engaged. The main "words" in this language are:

Tip (Angulation): This is the tooth's "nod." It controls the front-to-back tilt of the crown. Think of it as ensuring each tooth gives a friendly, properly angled greeting to the tooth next to it.

Torque (Inclination): This is the tooth's "posture." It dictates the crucial front-to-back lean of the entire tooth, from root to crown. Proper torque ensures the front teeth don't flare out or look too upright, giving the smile stability and a natural aesthetic.

In-Out: This ensures no tooth in the arch is "shy" (sitting too far back) or "bold" (jutting too far forward). The varying thickness of the bracket base helps create a smooth, flowing curve, like dancers perfectly aligned on a stage.

Over the years, different orthodontic visionaries have refined this language, creating unique prescriptions like Roth, MBT, and Alexander. These aren't competing systems so much as different dialects, each with its own nuances based on a philosophy of what creates the most stable, functional, and beautiful result.

The Dance of Force and Memory: How it All Works

The true magic happens in the elegant dance between the bracket and the archwire.

Imagine a brand-new, perfectly straight archwire. It's crafted from a special "memory" alloy, like nickel-titanium. Its one desire in life is to be straight.

Now, an orthodontist threads this wire through the newly placed brackets on a patient's crooked teeth. To fit into each bracket's pre-angled slot, the memory wire must bend and contort. It is now holding tension, a stored memory of its original, perfect form.

And so, the dance begins.

The wire, ever so gently, begins to pull itself straight again. As it does, it exerts a light, continuous force on the bracket. The bracket, bonded securely, transfers this silent instruction to the tooth. The tooth, responding to this persistent, gentle nudge, begins to move. It tips, it rotates, it torques through the bone, guided inexorably along the path the wire dictates. This continues until, one by one, each tooth moves into a position where its bracket slot is perfectly aligned with the wire.

When the wire is finally straight again, its work is done. The tooth has arrived at its pre-programmed destination.

The Artist is Still the Master

It would be a mistake to think this system turned orthodontists into mere technicians. The opposite is true. It freed them to focus on the bigger picture. The straight-wire system is a powerful instrument, but an instrument is only as good as the musician playing it.

The orthodontist's skill is more critical than ever. The precise placement of each bracket is paramount—an error of a fraction of a millimeter can change the final result. Their diagnosis of the underlying problem, their selection of the sequence of wires (from light and flexible to strong and rigid), and their management of the bite with tools like rubber bands are what elevate the process from a mechanical exercise to a life-changing treatment.

While new technologies like clear aligners have emerged, the principles uncovered by the straight-wire philosophy remain the bedrock of modern orthodontics. It taught us the very grammar of how to move teeth predictably and safely. It transformed the art of the smile from a handcrafted sculpture into an architectural masterpiece, built on a foundation of brilliant insight, elegant mechanics, and enduring clinical skill.

Beyond the Blueprint: Crafting Your One-of-a-Kind Smile

For years, getting braces was a bit like buying a beautiful, off-the-rack suit. The "straight-wire" system, a brilliant innovation in its own right, was designed for an "average" person. It fits most people pretty well, but it's never a truly custom fit. The brackets and wires have a standard prescription built in, assuming everyone's teeth, roots, and jaws are more or less the same.

But you're not average. Your body is a unique landscape. The curve of your jaw, the tilt of your roots, the very density of the bone holding your teeth are all yours alone. Relying on an average can mean a longer treatment time, unexpected detours, and a result that's good, but not perfectly you. The goal has shifted from simply straightening teeth to engineering a smile that is in perfect harmony with your individual biology. This is where the real magic begins.

Your Smile's Flight Simulator

So, how do we map this unique landscape? We use a technology straight out of the world of high-stakes engineering: Finite Element Analysis (FEA). Imagine an aerospace engineer designing a new jet. They don't just build it and hope it flies. They build a digital version first and run thousands of simulations, testing the wings against turbulence and the fuselage against pressure. They find every point of stress and every potential weakness before a single piece of metal is cut.

That's exactly what FEA does for your smile. It's a biomedical flight simulator for your teeth. Instead of experimenting in your mouth—which is, after all, a one-way trip—your orthodontist can run countless "what-if" scenarios in a completely safe, virtual space. It allows them to see exactly how your teeth will respond to different forces, predicting the outcome with incredible accuracy. It's a glimpse into the future of your treatment, ensuring the smoothest possible journey.

Building Your Digital Double

The process starts by creating your "digital double," an incredibly precise 3D model of you. This isn't a generic cartoon; it's a patient-specific masterpiece.

It all begins with advanced imaging. A Cone Beam Computed Tomography (CBCT) scan gives us a breathtakingly clear, three-dimensional view of your jawbones and tooth roots—the hidden architecture that supports your smile. Then, a comfortable Intraoral Scanner (IOS) painlessly maps the surfaces of your teeth and gums, capturing every unique contour.

These two data streams are then fused together, creating a comprehensive 3D model that is uniquely yours. This digital twin includes the precise shape of every tooth, the delicate network of ligaments (the Periodontal Ligament or PDL) that acts as a cushion, and the specific landscape of your bone. This ligament is the key—it's the communication channel where the physical forces of orthodontics are translated into the biological process of tooth movement.

The Virtual Design Studio

With your digital double loaded into the software, your orthodontist becomes less of a technician and more of an architect. In this virtual studio, they can place virtual brackets, test different types of wires, or design the perfect clear aligner.

They then apply a simulated force—the gentle, consistent pressure that will guide your teeth into their new positions. The FEA software then works its magic, running complex calculations to reveal a color-coded map of stress and tension across your digital jaw. It shows exactly how the forces travel through the tooth, into the ligament, and out to the surrounding bone.

Most importantly, the simulation predicts the exact initial movement of the tooth. It's not a guess; it's a prediction based on your specific anatomy and the precise forces being applied. This allows the orthodontist to refine the plan, making tiny adjustments to achieve the most efficient and healthy movement possible.

From Lab to Clinic: The 2025 Reality

This isn't science fiction. As of 2025, FEA is a real-world tool that's transforming orthodontic clinics.

It's being used to create truly custom appliances. For a particularly stubborn tooth, an orthodontist can design a unique bracket or attachment, engineered specifically for the job, ensuring the force is just right. For clear aligner wearers, FEA helps optimize the shape and placement of attachments—the small bumps that give the aligner the grip it needs—to execute complex movements with precision.

FEA also gives clinicians a superpower: the ability to compare futures. If there are a few different ways to approach your treatment, your orthodontist can simulate them all. They can virtually "test drive" each plan, compare the predicted outcomes side-by-side, and choose the path that is safest, fastest, and most effective for you. This foresight eliminates surprises and empowers you with the confidence that you're on the absolute best path.

A New Conversation with Your Smile

The power of FEA is in the questions it allows us to answer before we even begin. Your orthodontist can now ask the model:

"If we apply this gentle pressure to this specific canine, what is its exact path of movement? Will it tip or rotate in a way we don't want?"

"This patient's premolar has a unique shape. How can we design a force system to move the entire tooth—root and all—in perfect unison?"

This ability to rehearse and perfect the treatment on a digital double is the hallmark of modern orthodontics. It's a shift from a reactive to a proactive approach, saving you time in the chair and leading to a more predictable, successful outcome.

The Shift: From Following a Map to Drawing It

The arrival of FEA marks a profound change in orthodontics. We are moving away from a prescriptive world, where treatment was based on established rules and population averages, and into a predictive one.

Orthodontics has always been a blend of science and art. FEA doesn't remove the artistry; it enhances it with an unprecedented layer of engineering precision. By designing and validating your treatment in a virtual space first, your orthodontist can ensure that your journey to a new smile is not just based on experience, but is meticulously engineered for your unique biology. This is the new promise of orthodontics: a truly personal, predictable, and brilliant smile, designed just for you.

The Orthodontist's Dilemma: A Tale of Two Paths to a Perfect Smile

Every smile tells a story. Sometimes, it's a story with a few crooked characters or unexpected gaps in the plot. Straightening out that story is the art and science of orthodontics. But how do we guide those teeth into a beautiful, harmonious alignment? It's not about brute force; it's about a deep understanding of movement, a conversation between the orthodontist's tools and the body's own wisdom. At the heart of this process lies a fundamental choice, a fork in the road of treatment: do we slide or do we dance?

This is the choice between two profound strategies: the well-trodden path of frictional mechanics and the intricate choreography of frictionless mechanics. Choosing the right path is everything—it defines the journey, the comfort, and the brilliance of the final result.

The Grind: A Tooth's Journey on the Frictional Railway

Imagine your teeth are on a cross-country train trip. Each tooth has a tiny station—the bracket—and the journey happens along a single, continuous railway: the archwire. This is the world of frictional mechanics, the most common route in orthodontics. To close a gap, we essentially tell one tooth-train, "Time to move down the line and meet your neighbor." It sounds simple, and for many, it's an effective way to travel.

But have you ever tried to push a heavy box across a gritty floor? That stubborn, dragging resistance you feel? That's friction. In orthodontics, it's the invisible antagonist of this journey. This "drag" is a gremlin in the machine, an unpredictable force that builds up as the bracket grinds along the wire. It's caused by everything from the texture of a ceramic bracket to the very rubber band tying the wire in place.

Because of this constant resistance, the journey can become sluggish. To get things moving again, an orthodontist might have to give a bigger "push." But a bigger push isn't always a better one. This is where the concept of "anchorage" comes into play, and it's critical. Think of your anchor teeth as the strong, burly friends holding a rope while you try to pull something heavy. If you pull too hard, you don't just move the object; you drag your friends through the mud with you. In the mouth, this "anchorage loss" means the teeth you're relying on for stability start to move, too, creating a cascade of unwanted shifts. It's a classic case of one step forward, half a step back.

This is why we've seen the innovation of self-ligating brackets—the ones with a tiny, built-in gate to hold the wire. They were designed to be the "low-resistance" upgrade to the railway, aiming to let the train glide more freely. While they help, the fundamental challenge of the slide remains. Frictional mechanics is the powerful workhorse of orthodontics, but it's a path that requires navigating the constant, gritty reality of resistance.

The Dance: The Art of Frictionless Precision

Now, let's leave the railway behind and step into a dance studio. This is the world of frictionless mechanics. Here, there is no sliding, no dragging, no grinding. Instead, the orthodontist becomes a wire artist, a choreographer of movement.

The archwire is no longer a straight track but a canvas for intricate, custom designs. The orthodontist bends specific, elegant loops and springs into the wire—a "T-loop" here, a "closing loop" there. These aren't just for show; they are tiny, intelligent engines of force. When placed in the mouth, these activated loops and bends deliver a whisper-light, exquisitely precise push or pull, directly where it's needed.

Because there's no sliding, the gremlin of friction is banished. This is a game-changer. Without that resistance, the forces can be incredibly gentle and constant. They work in harmony with the body's natural rhythm of bone remodeling, coaxing teeth into place rather than coercing them. This biological "conversation" means less discomfort for the patient and a healthier, more stable result.

This method, however, demands immense skill. It's the difference between a pre-packaged meal and a gourmet dish crafted from scratch. The orthodontist must have the hands of a sculptor and the mind of an engineer, meticulously shaping the wire to express a specific movement. In its most advanced form, called "segmented arch mechanics," the wire is divided into independent parts. One segment acts as an unshakeable anchor, while another, armed with a delicate spring, performs a solo dance, guiding a single tooth or a small group with breathtaking precision. It's the method of choice for the most complex ballets—closing large gaps from extractions or guiding a rogue, impacted tooth back into the spotlight without disturbing its neighbors.

The Crystal Ball: Seeing the Smile Before It Happens

In this modern age, how does an orthodontist choose with confidence? Enter Finite Element Analysis (FEA), a tool that is nothing short of a digital crystal ball.

Imagine a stunningly detailed 3D model of your unique dental universe—every tooth, root, and bone structure mapped onto a computer. With FEA, we can stage a full dress rehearsal of your treatment. We can simulate the frictional railway and watch where the drag builds up. We can digitally test the higher forces and predict if your anchor teeth might start to slip.

Then, we can switch to the frictionless dance. We can design a virtual loop, apply its gentle force, and watch the tooth glide gracefully into its final position on the screen. FEA allows us to compare the two journeys side-by-side, revealing the hidden stresses, predicting the efficiency of movement, and mapping out the most comfortable, effective, and predictable path for you. It transforms the orthodontist's plan from an educated guess into a data-driven masterpiece.

A Personalized Masterpiece

In the end, the debate isn't about which method is "best," but which story we are trying to tell. Frictional mechanics is the powerful and straightforward prose for many of life's simpler narratives. Frictionless mechanics is the nuanced poetry reserved for the most intricate and challenging tales.

The true master orthodontist is bilingual, fluent in both the language of the slide and the art of the dance. They know when to rely on the steadfast railway and when to choreograph a delicate ballet of wires. By blending these techniques and peering into the future with tools like FEA, they can craft a treatment that is not just a technical procedure, but a personalized journey—one that ends with the beautiful, healthy, and confident smile you were always meant to have.

Part II: Managing Malocclusion in the Growing Patient

Adolescent Orthodontics: Navigating Growth and Development

The Sculptor and the River: Why Your Child's Growth Isn't Just a Phase—It's an Opportunity

Think of an orthodontist not as a mechanic for teeth, but as a sculptor. And their medium isn't clay or stone; it's the living, breathing, dynamic face of a growing child. This isn't just about straightening what's already there. It's about partnering with one of the most powerful forces in nature—the force of growth itself—to guide a masterpiece into being.

Imagine a young person's face as a river, its path slowly carved by the deep currents of genetics. For years, it flows along, shaping the landscape of their profile. But there are moments, incredible windows in time, when this river surges with power. During these brief, magical seasons, the banks are soft, and the current is malleable. A skilled guide can step in, not to dam the river, but to gently nudge its flow into a more harmonious, balanced channel. This is the art and science of craniofacial growth, and it's the secret behind truly life-changing orthodontic care.

A Tale of Two Jaws: The Steady Stream and the Wild River

Every face is a landscape dominated by two powerful jaws, and the key is knowing they move at entirely different rhythms.

The Upper Jaw (Maxilla): The Steady Stream. Like a river that carves its main path early, the upper jaw does most of its growing business sooner rather than later. It flows forward and down with a predictable current, establishing much of the facial foundation in early childhood. Its course can be influenced, but its primary journey is a steady, early one.

The Lower Jaw (Mandible): The Wild River. The lower jaw is a different story altogether. It's the late bloomer, the wilder current that meanders for a while before surging with incredible force during the teenage years. It is in this powerful, late-breaking rush of growth that an orthodontist finds their greatest opportunity. For a child whose lower jaw seems to lag behind, this is the golden moment to encourage it forward, to help it find its rightful, confident place in the world.

Watching over this entire landscape is the silent, steadfast cranial base—the ancient bedrock of the skull. It changes very little, providing the perfect, stable point from which to measure the incredible, dynamic journey of the jaws below.

The Golden Tide: Riding the Wave of Puberty

If growth is a river, then the pubertal growth spurt is the golden tide. It's a massive, hormone-fueled wave of development that floods the entire system. During this window, everything is in flux. Bone isn't a static scaffold; it's a vibrant, buzzing hub of cellular energy, ready and willing to be influenced.

This is the orthodontist's moment.

This is when a special device, like a "functional appliance," can act as a gentle guide. For a child with a recessed lower jaw, this appliance doesn't use brute force. It whispers to the body. By posturing the jaw slightly forward, it sends a biological signal to the growth centers, saying, "A little more length right here would be perfect." The body, already in high-growth mode, listens and responds. It's a beautiful, biological conversation—a dance between gentle intervention and nature's powerful intent.

To miss this tide is to be left on the shore. Once the surge of puberty recedes, the bone hardens, the riverbanks firm up, and the window for this profound, natural change slams shut. What could have been achieved with a gentle nudge may now require more extensive camouflage or even future surgery.

Reading the Body's Secret Language

So, how does an orthodontist know when this golden tide is about to roll in? They become expert trackers, learning to read the body's secret language. This isn't about age; it's about developmental timing.

They might look at a side-view x-ray of the head, focusing not on the teeth, but on the changing shapes of the vertebrae in the neck. These bones mature in a predictable sequence, acting as a secret code that reveals, "The spurt is beginning," "We are at its peak," or "The major growth is complete." They watch a child's height skyrocket on a growth chart. They observe the other tell-tale signs of puberty. By piecing together these clues, they can pinpoint the perfect time to act.

The Shape of Your Flow: Vertical vs. Horizontal

Beyond when growth happens, there's the critical question of which way it's headed.

Some faces grow like a waterfall, with a strong downward, or vertical, motion. This can lead to a longer facial profile and a bite where the front teeth struggle to meet. The orthodontist's goal here is to gently redirect this vertical cascade, promoting harmony and balance.

Other faces grow like a powerful forward current, or horizontally. This can result in a shorter lower face and a deep, overlapping bite. Here, the art is to encourage a bit more of that gentle, vertical dimension to soften the profile and create a more balanced result.

Identifying this innate pattern is like understanding the prevailing wind before setting sail. You don't fight it; you harness it. You work with the natural flow of the face to create a result that is not only beautiful but will last a lifetime because it is in harmony with the body's own design.

A Partnership with Your Potential

In the end, this deep understanding transforms orthodontics from a mechanical procedure into a biological art form. It's about seeing the incredible, untapped potential locked within every young person's growth. When an orthodontist times their intervention to perfectly sync with the body's own powerful growth spurt, something truly special happens.

The result is more than a straight smile. It's a balanced profile, a healthy function, and a radiant confidence that comes from a face that was gently guided to its full, spectacular potential. It's the art of revealing the masterpiece that was always waiting to emerge.

The Secret Clockwork of a Child's Smile: Why Your Age is Just a Number

How old is your child? Ten? Thirteen? It's a simple question with a surprisingly complex answer, especially when it comes to a journey as important as creating a healthy, confident smile. We tend to think of age as a straightforward number, a line neatly drawn from one birthday to the next. But in the world of growth and development, this "chronological age" is more of a suggestion than a rule.

Imagine two thirteen-year-olds standing side-by-side. One might be on the cusp of a major growth spurt, their body a coiled spring of potential. The other might still be a few years away from that same burst of energy. They share a number, but their internal, biological clocks are telling completely different stories. For an orthodontist, listening to this hidden clock is everything. Relying on just a birthdate to plan treatment is like trying to catch a train using a calendar instead of a timetable. You might get lucky, but more often than not, you'll miss the perfect moment.

This is where the art and science of skeletal maturity come in, a way to listen to the body's own timetable and pinpoint the "golden hour" for growth.

Reading the Bones: A Story Written in the Hand

For decades, the most trusted method for tuning into this biological clock was a simple X-ray of the hand and wrist. It might seem odd—peering into the hand to understand the jaw—but it was a stroke of genius. The hand is a bustling city of small bones, each on its own schedule of transformation. This process, called ossification, is like watching a sculptor slowly turn soft cartilage into hard, defined bone.

An experienced eye can look at a hand-wrist X-ray and see a story unfolding. Are the bones still like soft, rounded pebbles? Or have they sharpened, defined their edges, and begun to fuse together in a predictable, elegant dance? Each stage is a chapter in the tale of a child's growth. It's a beautifully accurate method, revealing a "skeletal age" that speaks volumes more than a birth certificate ever could. It's like looking at a tree's rings; the number of rings tells you its age, but their thickness and character tell you the story of its seasons—its periods of drought and its moments of vibrant growth.

But this classic method, for all its wisdom, came with a catch. It required its own, separate X-ray. In a world where we've become rightly conscious of every bit of radiation exposure, adding an extra procedure, no matter how small, gave us pause. Coupled with the extra time and cost, the search was on for a more streamlined way to get the same crucial information.

The Spine's Secret: A Code Hiding in Plain Sight

The breakthrough came from looking at an X-ray that was already a routine part of every orthodontic visit: the lateral cephalometric radiograph. This is the classic side-profile X-ray that helps orthodontists map out the landscape of the jaw and skull. For years, we had the answer right in front of us, a secret code hiding in plain sight within the elegant curve of the neck.

This is the Cervical Vertebral Maturation (CVM) method. It focuses on just three small bones in the neck—the second, third, and fourth cervical vertebrae (C2, C3, and C4). As a child navigates the rapids of puberty and its powerful growth spurts, these vertebrae undergo a fascinating and reliable transformation. Early on, they have a delicate, wedge-like shape. As the growth engine roars to life, they begin to stretch and become more rectangular. Finally, as the growth spurt winds down, they settle into a more solid, square form.

This predictable sequence is a built-in biological GPS. By simply observing the shape of these three little bones on an X-ray that was going to be taken anyway, an orthodontist can see exactly where a patient is on their growth journey. No extra X-ray. No added radiation. No additional cost. It was a paradigm shift, allowing us to unlock vital information with elegant efficiency.

Enter the Oracle: AI and the Future of the Perfect Smile

Now, we are stepping into an even more exciting era, one where we partner human expertise with the incredible power of Artificial Intelligence. Think of an AI not as a replacement for an orthodontist, but as a super-powered assistant with flawless memory and boundless experience. These AI algorithms are trained on tens of thousands of X-rays, learning to see the subtle, almost invisible, patterns of growth.

The true magic of AI is its objectivity. Even the most skilled human eye can have slight variations in judgment. An orthodontist might interpret an X-ray slightly differently on a Monday morning versus a Friday afternoon. AI eliminates this human variable. It applies the same precise, data-driven analysis every single time, offering a level of standardization and consistency we've never had before. Studies show its incredible promise, with accuracy rates in CVM analysis climbing as high as 90%, and even higher when analyzing the traditional hand-wrist X-rays.

This technology is doing more than just speeding things up; it's deepening our understanding. An AI can analyze an image in a fraction of a second, providing quantifiable data that supports and enhances the orthodontist's clinical judgment.

The Human Element: Where Biology Meets Biography

This brings us to the most important part of the entire story. The most advanced AI, the most precise biological data, is only one half of the equation. The other half is the patient. The perfect treatment window isn't just a biological event; it's a human one.

This is the concept of psychosocial readiness. Is the child mature enough to understand the commitment? Are they motivated to keep their braces clean and handle the responsibilities of treatment? Does the family have the support system in place to navigate the journey?

The ultimate success of orthodontic care lies at the beautiful intersection where a child's biological readiness meets their personal readiness. AI-powered analysis gives us an unprecedented, crystal-clear view of the biological green light. It tells us, with stunning precision, that the body is ready to be gently guided toward its ideal form.

Our job, then, is to place this powerful insight into the context of a real child's life. When we can align that perfect biological timing with a patient who is motivated, ready, and excited for their transformation, the results are more than just straight teeth. We create a positive, empowering experience that leads to a lifetime of confident, healthy smiles. It's a partnership between the oracle of data and the heart of the individual, crafting the perfect outcome, one unique child at a time.

The Architecture of a Smile: Solving the Puzzles of the Bite

Straight teeth are only half the story. The true magic of a brilliant smile lies in its architecture—the way the upper and lower jaws meet, the way the teeth fit together in a perfect, harmonious puzzle. But what happens when the puzzle pieces don't quite fit? In the world of growing smiles, orthodontists often play the role of master architects, solving two of the most common and fascinating structural challenges: the deep bite and the open bite.

These aren't just cosmetic quirks. They are vertical discrepancies, meaning the height and overlap of the front teeth are off-kilter. Tackling these issues during the adolescent growth spurt is like working with pliable clay—it's the golden window to guide the jaws and teeth into a design that is not only beautiful but built to last a lifetime.

The Vanishing Lower Teeth: Cracking the Case of the Deep Bite

Imagine a curtain call where the front curtain drops so low it completely hides the performers on stage. This is a deep bite. When someone with a deep bite closes their mouth, their upper front teeth descend like a veil, almost completely covering the lower front teeth. In more serious cases, those lower teeth can even bite into the sensitive gum tissue on the roof of the mouth.

The Blueprint of a Deep Bite

So, what causes this? Often, it's a story of growth direction. Picture a face that grows more forward than downward, creating a shorter, more compact facial profile. As the lower jaw grows, it can rotate slightly upward and forward, like a closing drawbridge that swings a little too far shut.

This action nudges the lower front teeth deeper behind the uppers.

Sometimes the teeth themselves are the culprits. Overeager front teeth might erupt too far, while back teeth remain shy, not erupting enough to prop the bite open. Even the body's own power can be a factor. Immensely strong chewing muscles can press the back teeth down, like weights holding them in place, further deepening the bite in the front.

Why It's More Than Just a Look

A deep bite can be a silent saboteur. The most immediate threat is to the teeth themselves. The relentless pressure and friction can wear down the enamel on the lower front teeth, stripping them of their protective coating. It can also trap the lower jaw, limiting the easy side-to-side movements we need for efficient chewing. And the constant irritation to the gums can lead to soreness, inflammation, and recession.

Classic Tools for Leveling the Foundation

For generations, orthodontists have used ingenious methods to re-level this bite. The goal is simple: get the back teeth to grow taller or gently nudge the front teeth back into their proper place.

One classic hero is the anterior bite plate. This small, custom-made acrylic shelf sits discreetly behind the upper front teeth. When the patient bites, the lower teeth hit this plate, which acts like a doorstop, preventing the front bite from closing all the way. This simple act liberates the back teeth, giving them the space to erupt naturally into a taller, more stable position, which in turn levels out the front.

Another approach uses the physics of specialized wires. A reverse curve of Spee wire, for example, is shaped like a subtle smile. When snapped into the braces, it applies a gentle, upward push on the front teeth while simultaneously encouraging the back teeth to erupt downward—a brilliant two-for-one move to flatten and open the bite. These time-tested methods are clever and effective, but they rely heavily on a patient's natural growth and, in the case of removable plates, unwavering cooperation.

The Unfinished Bridge: The Challenge of the Anterior Open Bite

Now, let's flip the script. Imagine a bridge where the two ends never quite meet, leaving a persistent gap in the middle. This is an anterior open bite. When a person bites down on their back teeth, their front teeth—both upper and lower—don't touch. This gap can make simple acts, like biting into a slice of pizza, a frustrating impossibility.

The Troublemakers Behind the Gap

Open bites are often a more complex mystery with several potential culprits:

A Downward Spiral: The most common cause is a skeletal growth pattern where the back of the upper jaw grows excessively downward. This over-eruption of the back molars acts like a pivot, causing the lower jaw to swing down and back. This rotation hinges the bite open at the front, often creating a longer facial appearance.

The Habit Saboteurs: Persistent habits are powerful forces. A thumb or finger that lingers in the mouth past early childhood can physically block the front teeth from erupting and push them out of alignment. The tongue thrust is another major player—a rebellious habit where the tongue pushes forward between the teeth during swallowing. This constant, gentle pressure is enough to keep the teeth apart, creating and maintaining an open bite.

The Airway Connection: Chronic mouth breathing, often due to enlarged tonsils or allergies, forces the tongue to abandon its rightful post on the roof of the mouth. A low-lying tongue fails to shape the upper jaw correctly and often develops a thrusting habit to create an oral seal, compounding the problem.

Why an Open Bite Matters

Functionally, an open bite is a daily frustration. It impacts speech, sometimes causing lisps, and turns eating into a chore. Aesthetically, the visible gap can be a source of self-consciousness, dimming the light of a person's smile.

Traditional Attempts to Close the Gap

Historically, the mission was to stop the back teeth from erupting further. High-pull headgear was a common tool—a device using straps over the head to apply an upward force to the upper molars. The goal was to halt their downward growth and encourage the jaw to rotate closed. But this required a heroic level of patient cooperation, often 12-14 hours of wear a day.

Posterior bite blocks, either fixed or removable, were another strategy. These acrylic pads sit on top of the back teeth, physically preventing them from erupting and sometimes encouraging the front teeth to move toward each other. While these methods could work, they were often a slow battle against powerful growth patterns and dependent on a patient's commitment.

The Revolution: Micro-Anchors and the Power of TADs

The story of vertical correction was dramatically rewritten with the arrival of Temporary Anchorage Devices (TADs). These aren't appliances; they're tiny, biocompatible titanium screws that act as rock-solid, temporary anchor points in the bone. They are the orthodontist's secret weapon, providing an unmovable object to push or pull against.

The Magic of Absolute Anchorage

In traditional orthodontics, moving one tooth requires bracing against another. It's like trying to push a car while standing on a skateboard—you're likely to move backward yourself. TADs are like standing on solid ground. Placed directly into the bone, they don't budge, allowing for incredibly precise and efficient tooth movement without any unwanted side effects.

TADs: The Open Bite's Greatest Foe

This is where TADs truly shine. For severe, skeletal open bites, they are nothing short of revolutionary.

The Setup: In a quick and minor procedure, TADs are placed in the bone of the upper jaw, typically above the back molars.

The Force: The orthodontist then attaches tiny elastic chains from these micro-anchors directly to the molars.

The Miracle of Intrusion: This creates a direct, constant, upward force that gently pushes the over-erupted molars back up into the jawbone.

This molar intrusion is the key that unlocks the entire system. As the back of the bite moves up, the lower jaw is free to rotate upward and forward—like a drawbridge smoothly closing. This single, powerful movement brings the front teeth together, closing the open bite in a way that is more predictable, efficient, and less dependent on patient compliance than ever before.

It Takes a Village to Build a Smile

Even with revolutionary technology, lasting success comes from a holistic view. It's a team effort.

Habit Whispering: For open bites, breaking a thumb-sucking or tongue-thrusting habit is non-negotiable. This may involve behavioral therapy or specialized "reminder" appliances.

Muscle Re-education: A myofunctional therapist can work wonders, retraining the tongue to rest and swallow correctly, creating a stable internal environment for the teeth.

Clearing the Airway: If mouth breathing is the issue, collaborating with an ENT specialist to address enlarged tonsils or allergies can be a critical step.

The Guardian Retainer: After the architectural work is complete, retainers are the guardians that ensure the beautiful new structure remains stable for years to come.

In the end, managing vertical discrepancies is about more than just wires and brackets. It's about understanding the unique story of a patient's growth. With a blend of time-honored principles and groundbreaking innovations like TADs, orthodontists can solve these complex puzzles, building functional, breathtaking smiles that are truly engineered for life.

The Unspoken Contract: A Smile is More Than Straight Teeth

Orthodontic treatment is a silent agreement. On one side, there's the science—the precise angles, the gentle pressures, the elegant dance of biomechanics that nudges teeth into their rightful places. On the other, there's the human heart of the equation: the teenager in the chair. And without their willing partnership, the most brilliant blueprint for a perfect smile is just an idea on a chart.

This is the central truth, the one that modern, empathetic orthodontics is built upon. It's why pioneering programs, like the one at Saint Louis University, insist on teaching "Child and Adolescent Psychology." They know that we aren't just treating a bite; we are caring for a person during one of the most turbulent and defining chapters of their life.

Navigating the Adolescent Storm

Think of adolescence as a renovation of the self. Everything is under construction. Teenagers are drafting the blueprints of their own identity, trying on different versions of who they want to be. Their social world becomes the primary stage, and the spotlight of peer opinion feels incredibly bright and often harsh. Their relationship with their own reflection is complicated, a daily negotiation with an ever-changing body. And above all, they are filled with a fierce, burgeoning desire for independence—to be the architects of their own lives.

Now, into this whirlwind, introduce orthodontic treatment. It's not a simple medical fix. It's an intrusion. It's a public project happening right in the center of their face, impacting how they look, how they feel, and how they navigate their social lives. Understanding this isn't just a courtesy; it's the key to unlocking success.

The Three Sparks: What Truly Powers the Journey

Beneath the surface of every orthodontic journey, three emotional currents are at play: motivation, compliance, and self-esteem. They are deeply intertwined, each one feeding—or starving—the others.

Motivation: The 'Why' Behind the Wires

Motivation is the quiet engine that drives the whole process. It's the difference between a patient who is a passenger and one who is a co-pilot.

The Fire Within (Intrinsic Motivation): This is the gold standard. It's the teen who has a personal vision for their future smile. Maybe they've felt the sting of a cruel joke, or perhaps they simply hold a clear picture of a more confident self. This inner resolve is what fuels them to brush meticulously around every bracket, to pop their elastics in without being reminded, to say "no" to the gummy candies that could derail their progress. The goal is theirs, and that ownership changes everything.

The Gentle Nudge (Extrinsic Motivation): This is the push from the outside world—the desire to make parents happy, the promise of a reward, or the wish to simply get the whole process over with. While it can kickstart the journey, it's like running on battery power. It eventually fades. A teen who feels like they're wearing braces for someone else will likely offer just enough cooperation to get by, leading to a rockier, longer road with compromised results.

The true art of orthodontics, then, is to become a kind of motivational alchemist, helping to transform the external nudge into a genuine internal fire.

Compliance: Turning Intention into Action

Compliance is where the rubber meets the road—or, more accurately, where the elastic meets the bracket. It's the daily, often tedious, translation of motivation into tangible habits. Wearing elastics for 20-plus hours, choosing the right foods, keeping a complex architecture of metal and wires spotlessly clean—these aren't small asks for a teenager juggling school, friends, and a rapidly changing life.

When we see compliance falter, it's rarely defiance. It's the chaotic reality of being a teenager. They forget. They get swept up in the moment. They crave the forbidden pizza crust. A compassionate approach understands this. It's not about wagging a finger; it's about finding a way to make the right choice the easier, more understood choice.

Self-Esteem: The Face in the Mirror

Nowhere is the adolescent experience more fragile than in the realm of self-esteem. The mirror can be a friend or a foe, and body image is a constant internal dialogue. For some, braces can feel like a social setback, a highly visible symbol of imperfection in a world that worships flawlessness.

This is where the evolution of orthodontic technology has been nothing short of a revolution in kindness. The shift from a one-size-fits-all approach of metal braces to a menu of more subtle options is transformative. Tooth-colored ceramic braces that whisper rather than shout, or clear aligners that are practically a secret between the patient and their orthodontist, empower the teenager. They diminish the feeling of being a "metal mouth," allowing their confidence to breathe and grow even while their smile is still a work in progress.

The Orthodontist Reimagined: More Than a Clinician

The modern orthodontist must wear many hats, and "wire-bender" is only the beginning. They must become a trusted guide on a very personal journey.

As a Coach: A great coach doesn't just bark orders from the sidelines. They inspire, they explain the strategy behind the play, and they celebrate every small yard gained. They build a partnership by explaining the "why," setting clear and honest expectations, and reminding the patient that the temporary discomfort is a stepping stone to a permanent victory.

As an Educator: The goal is to translate complex instructions into a language a teenager can hear and absorb. It's about showing, not just telling. It's about framing the consequences of non-compliance not as threats, but as simple, unavoidable truths: "If the elastics aren't worn, the teeth won't move. It's a law of physics, and we're in this together to make it work."

As an Empath: This is the most crucial role. It means creating a space where a teenager feels safe to be vulnerable. It's about listening to their frustrations about a poking wire or their anxiety about school pictures. It's about validating their feelings and respecting their growing need for autonomy by including them in decisions. When a patient feels seen and heard, they don't just comply; they engage.

The Ripple Effect: A Legacy of Confidence

When all these human elements align with the clinical science, something magical happens. The result isn't just a set of straight teeth. It's a profound and lasting transformation. A beautiful smile becomes a gateway to newfound confidence that can ripple through every aspect of a young person's life—their willingness to raise their hand in class, their courage to try out for the play, their ease in meeting new people.

They also gain a deep-seated understanding of their own health and the rewards of discipline and partnership. This patient-centered journey, this holistic and human approach, turns a medical necessity into an empowering rite of passage. It delivers not just a corrected bite, but a more resilient, confident, and radiant human being, ready to share their smile with the world.

Non-Extraction and Extraction Protocols: A Profile-Driven, Evidence-Based Approach

Behind every confident smile lies a hidden history, a quiet war of ideas fought not with armies, but with wires, brackets, and profoundly different visions of human beauty. The landscape of modern orthodontics, where your treatment is as unique as your fingerprint, was carved from a century-long clash between two titans—a visionary artist and a pragmatic engineer—who forever changed the shape of the human face.

The Architect of Perfection: Dr. Angle's 32-Pillar Temple

At the dawn of the 20th century, Dr. Edward Angle, the undisputed father of orthodontics, saw the human mouth as a sacred temple. He was an idealist, a purist who believed nature's design was flawless. His gospel was simple and profound: all 32 teeth, every last one, was a non-negotiable pillar in this perfect architectural system. To him, a misaligned smile wasn't a sign of having too many teeth, but of a foundation—the dental arch—that hadn't been allowed to reach its magnificent, God-given potential.

His mission was one of expansion. Angle was the grand architect who would widen the temple grounds to make room for every pillar. His tools were designed to stretch and mold the jaw, creating a broader, more sweeping smile that could accommodate all 32 teeth in what he called "ideal occlusion"—a harmony so perfect, the teeth would fit together like the gears of a divine watch. Removing a tooth was more than a compromise; it was sacrilege. It was admitting that the blueprint was flawed, a betrayal of the natural perfection he so deeply revered. His philosophy was a siren song of idealism, and for a time, the entire profession sailed in his direction.

A Beautiful Theory's Ugly Secret

But reality, as it often does, had other plans. As a generation of orthodontists followed Angle's non-extraction doctrine, a troubling truth began to emerge from behind the braces. The perfect smiles weren't holding. Like a building on an unstable foundation, the teeth would begin to shift and crumble back toward their old, crooked positions in a heartbreaking process known as relapse.

Worse, the pursuit of this dental ideal was creating an unforeseen aesthetic problem. In trying to fit all 32 pillars onto a foundation that was simply too small, the front teeth were often shoved dramatically forward. This created a "full" or "protrusive" look, a facial profile that seemed to bulge around the mouth. Patients, promised a look of harmony, were left with strained lips stretched over a smile that felt too big for their face. Angle's beautiful theory, when applied universally, was creating outcomes that were neither stable nor, in many eyes, beautiful. The very bedrock of the jaw had limits, and the grand, 32-pillar temple simply couldn't be built on every landscape.

The Engineering Revolution: Charles Tweed's Calculated Sacrifice

From within Angle's own intellectual lineage came the rebellion. Dr. Charles Tweed, a brilliant student of the master, witnessed the collapsing smiles and strained faces firsthand. He was a pragmatist, an engineer who understood that a beautiful design is useless if it cannot stand the test of time. He realized that the problem wasn't the blueprint, but the failure to adapt it to the real-world limitations of the building site—the patient's own skeleton.

Tweed's counter-philosophy was a stroke of engineering genius born from painful observation. He argued that for a smile to be both beautiful and permanent, the teeth had to live comfortably within the natural boundary of their underlying bone. If the land was too small, you couldn't just keep building. His solution was revolutionary and, to the purists, heretical: strategic removal.

Typically, this meant removing four bicuspid teeth. This wasn't a surrender; it was a calculated sacrifice. This "controlled demolition" created the critical space needed to retract the front teeth, pulling them back from their forward-straining position into a profile of elegant balance. Tweed's goal wasn't just a straight smile, but a stable one that brought the lips, chin, and nose into a natural, unstrained harmony. He wasn't just fixing teeth; he was re-sculpting the face with the long-term reality of bone and biology as his guide.

The Pendulum of Battle

Tweed's ideas detonated a civil war within orthodontics. For decades, the profession became a battlefield of opposing ideals. The "non-extractionists" clung to Angle's vision of natural perfection, arguing that removing healthy teeth was a mutilation that could lead to other problems. The "extractionists" championed Tweed's realism, holding up their stable, aesthetically pleasing results as undeniable proof that less could, in fact, be more.

This was no dry academic debate. It was a passionate, deeply personal conflict over the very definition of a successful outcome. The pendulum of opinion swung violently back and forth with every new study and every charismatic leader. It was a crucible of innovation, forcing orthodontists to look deeper, question everything, and refine their craft under the pressure of intense disagreement.

Out of that fiery, century-long debate, the modern orthodontist was forged. Today's practitioner is no longer a disciple of one school, but a master of both. They are both artist and engineer, idealist and realist. They begin with Angle's reverence for the natural dentition but assess it with Tweed's critical, engineering eye. They understand that the perfect smile isn't a one-size-fits-all template, but a custom-built masterpiece, a synthesis of competing truths, designed to fit the unique and beautiful landscape of a single human face.

The Architect of the Smile: A New Blueprint for Orthodontic Decisions

In the quiet of the consultation room, a question hangs in the air, a pivotal crossroad in a person's journey to a new smile: "Will we need to pull teeth?"

For generations, the answer has rested in the hands of a skilled artisan—the orthodontist. More than a doctor, they are an architect of the face, a sculptor who sees not just teeth, but the delicate harmony of lips, chin, and profile. Their decision is a blend of science and soul, of learned principles and a seasoned artist's eye. It's a craft honed over thousands of cases, where they weigh the very architecture of a person's smile.

They hold the blueprints—the X-rays and molds—and begin their complex calculations. Is the foundation, the jaw, wide enough for the structures it must support? This is the classic dilemma of crowding, like having grand furniture for a small room. They examine the facade—the way the front teeth stand. Are they leaning forward, pushing the lips into a strained posture? Or are they tucked back, creating a flattened profile? They study the soft, living materials of the face, the lips and chin, understanding that moving a single tooth can change the entire landscape of a person's expression. And for the young, they become fortune-tellers, gazing into the future of a growing jaw, wondering if nature itself will lend a hand.

This has always been the way: a deeply personal analysis, a judgment call made by a trusted expert. But even the most brilliant architect is guided by their own experience, their own library of past projects. What if they could consult a global archive of every similar blueprint ever drawn, and see the final results of each one?

A Million Second Opinions in an Instant

This is the dawn of a new era, and it's powered by Artificial Intelligence. Don't picture a robot taking over the architect's chair. Instead, imagine a powerful new tool resting on the drafting table. AI is not a replacement for the orthodontist; it is their ultimate consultant, a co-pilot with a photographic memory of countless past journeys.

Think of it as a GPS for the smile. While a seasoned orthodontist navigates by the stars of their own experience, the AI has access to a satellite view of thousands upon thousands of successfully completed cases. It's been trained on an immense library of "before and after" stories. It has learned the subtle, almost invisible patterns that connect a patient's initial state to their final, radiant outcome.

How does it work its magic? The AI pores over the same blueprints the orthodontist uses, but with the tireless precision of a supercomputer.

It reads the language of cephalometrics—the complex angles and measurements on an X-ray that map the relationship between teeth, jaws, and skull. To the human eye, it's a series of numbers; to the AI, it's a detailed topographical map revealing hidden correlations.

It quantifies crowding with inhuman accuracy, calculating the tooth-to-arch-space discrepancy down to the micron. It analyzes facial photos, not just as a picture, but as a constellation of data points. It maps the curve of a lip, the angle of the nose, the projection of the chin, and cross-references these facial aesthetics with its vast database to see what has worked before.

After absorbing all this information, the AI does what it does best: it recognizes patterns. It sifts through its library of thousands of cases and finds the ones that look remarkably like the person sitting in the chair. It then presents its findings: "In cases with this specific combination of jaw structure, tooth alignment, and facial profile, 85% of the most successful, stable, and aesthetically pleasing outcomes were achieved by creating space without extractions." Or, conversely, it might advise that an extraction path led to a more balanced and harmonious result in similar situations.

With an accuracy reported between 80% and 93%, this isn't a guess. It's a data-driven forecast, an objective second opinion that cuts through habit and subjective bias.

The Human Touch in a Digital Age

This fusion of human artistry and machine intelligence is creating a revolution in care. It offers a new level of confidence and predictability. The conversation between orthodontist and patient can now be enriched with objective data, building trust and demystifying the treatment plan. It promises a future of more personalized medicine, where the proposed path is tailored not just to a general type of problem, but to a patient's unique structural and facial identity.

Of course, this powerful tool must be wielded with wisdom. The quality of the AI's advice is entirely dependent on the quality and diversity of the data it learns from. We must be vigilant against building biases into the system, ensuring its library of "successful cases" represents all faces and all people. The orthodontist's role becomes even more crucial, for they are the keepers of the human element.

The AI can analyze a blueprint, but it cannot understand a patient's hopes or fears. It can recommend a path, but it cannot offer a reassuring hand or share in the joy of the final reveal. The "why" behind the AI's recommendation—the so-called "black box"—still requires the interpretation and clinical judgment of an experienced professional who can look at the data, look at the patient, and make the final, human-centered decision.

The future of orthodontics isn't a world of algorithms and automation. It's a world of collaboration, where the architect's timeless wisdom is amplified by an extraordinary new instrument. It's a partnership that promises to make the journey to a new smile more efficient, more predictable, and more beautifully tailored to the individual than ever before. The art is not lost; it's simply being given a clearer, more detailed map to create its masterpiece.

The Smile Architect: A New Philosophy of Orthodontics

Your smile is your signature, a unique expression of who you are. For years, the path to a perfectly aligned smile often came with a difficult choice: removing healthy teeth to make room. It felt like a compromise, a sacrifice of the whole to perfect the parts. But what if there was a different way? What if, instead of demolition, we chose to be architects?

Welcome to the philosophy of non-extraction orthodontics. This isn't just a set of techniques; it's a belief that the most beautiful smile is a full one, one that works in harmony with your natural facial structure. It's a patient-centered approach that honors what you already have. An orthodontist embracing this path is like a master architect who, instead of tearing down walls, finds ingenious ways to expand, refine, and reimagine the space, creating a masterpiece that is both stunning and structurally sound.

They do this with a powerful toolkit designed not to subtract, but to create. Let's pull back the curtain on three of these modern marvels, each a testament to the art of creating space where none seems to exist.

1. Expansion: Raising the Cathedral Ceiling of Your Smile

Imagine your dental arch is a beautiful, vaulted room. If the room is too narrow, the furniture inside—your teeth—will be crowded and cramped. Expansion is the art of gently widening that room, of raising the cathedral ceiling to let the light in and give everything its proper place. It's about creating a broader, more breathtaking foundation for your smile.

How the Architecture is Redesigned:

For the Young Architect (Orthopedic Expansion): In children and teens, the upper jaw is like a blueprint still open to edits. It exists in two halves, joined by a soft seam. Using an appliance like a Palatal Expander, the orthodontist applies gentle, steady pressure, encouraging that seam to widen. It's a quiet miracle of biology; as the two halves separate, your own body fills the space with new bone. This isn't just moving teeth; it's fundamentally reshaping the architecture of the jaw, correcting crossbites and creating significant, lasting space for a smile to truly blossom.

For the Established Masterpiece (Dental Expansion): In adults, where the jaw's foundation is set, the focus shifts to elegantly rearranging the furniture. Here, expansion involves carefully tipping the teeth outward, angling them into a more ideal, spacious arc. Modern tools like Clear Aligners (e.g., Invisalign) are masters of this subtle art. Each aligner is a pre-designed step in a dance, coaxing the teeth into a wider, more harmonious arrangement.

Expansion is a foundational act of creation. It results in a full, radiant smile that complements the entire face. It's a commitment to a bigger picture, but one that requires a period of stabilization—like letting the foundation of a new building settle—to ensure the beautiful new dimensions last a lifetime.

2. Interproximal Reduction (IPR): The Art of the Whisper-Thin Space

Now, imagine the teeth are not furniture, but exquisitely carved sculptures standing side-by-side in a gallery. Sometimes, all that's needed for a perfect arrangement is for two sculptures to fit more intimately together. IPR is the delicate, precise art of polishing the sides where two teeth touch, removing a whisper-thin sliver of outer enamel—often no thicker than a piece of paper.

This isn't "stripping" or "filing" your teeth; it's the dental equivalent of a master gem-cutter faceting a diamond. By creating these minuscule spaces between several teeth, the orthodontist unlocks just enough room to resolve crowding, refine the shape of a tooth, or close those pesky "black triangles" that can sometimes appear at the gumline.

The Sculptor's Tools:

With the steady hand of an artist, an orthodontist uses fine, diamond-dusted strips or discs to gently polish the enamel. The surface is then smoothed and fortified, leaving it healthy and clean. It's a meticulous, controlled process that is the cornerstone of many clear aligner treatments, allowing for a level of perfection that was once unimaginable.

IPR is the art of subtlety. It proves that sometimes, the smallest, most precise changes can have the most profound impact, transforming a crowded arrangement into a seamless, flowing work of art.

3. Distalization: The Strategic Grand Retreat

Picture your teeth as dancers on a stage. If the stage is too crowded at the front, the solution isn't to remove dancers. It's to ask the back row to take a few steps upstage. Distalization is this strategic and graceful retreat. It's the process of moving your back teeth (the molars) further into the jaw to create a cascade of space at the front.

A Modern Choreography:

In the past, this movement often required bulky headgear, a cumbersome apparatus that relied entirely on you to do the work. Today's orthodontics has replaced that with elegant, unseen forces working behind the scenes.

Effortless Engines: Appliances like the Carriere Motion Appliance are like tiny, silent engines attached discreetly inside your mouth. They connect a back molar to a tooth further forward and exert a constant, gentle pressure, pushing the entire back segment of your teeth rearward. They work 24/7, no compliance needed, efficiently correcting your bite and creating space before braces or aligners even begin their work.

The Power of the Anchor: The true game-changer is the Temporary Anchorage Device (TAD). A TAD is a tiny, sterile anchor—no bigger than an earring stud—that is placed painlessly into the jawbone for a short time. This anchor provides an immovable point. From here, the orthodontist can use invisible forces to move only the specific teeth they want to move, with unparalleled precision. It's like a rock climber using a secure anchor to pull themselves up a cliff face; the TAD ensures all the force goes exactly where it's needed, preventing other teeth from shifting.

Distalization is a brilliant solution for creating significant space without extractions, especially for correcting overbites. It's a testament to how modern orthodontics can choreograph complex movements with grace and efficiency, leading to results that are both healthy and aesthetically spectacular.

A Smile, Whole and Complete

Choosing a non-extraction journey is choosing to believe in the wholeness of your smile. Through the architectural vision of Expansion, the sculptural precision of IPR, and the strategic choreography of Distalization, today's orthodontist can achieve what was once thought impossible: a perfectly aligned, fully functional, and radiantly complete smile, all without asking you to part with a single tooth. It's more than just straightening teeth—it's the art of revealing the masterpiece that was there all along.

The Smile Architect: A New Blueprint for Transformation

A smile is a story. Sometimes, it's a simple, elegant tale told in a straight line. Other times, the narrative is more complex, with characters crowded together, out of place, waiting for a guiding hand to bring them into harmony. For an orthodontist, the work is less about straightening teeth and more about becoming the architect of that story. And sometimes, to build something truly beautiful and lasting, you first have to make a difficult choice about the foundation.

This is the story of making space.

It's a decision that echoes with weight and care, a crossroad in the journey to a new smile: the decision to extract a tooth. This isn't a failure or a shortcut. It's a deliberate, thoughtful act of creation. Think of it not as a loss, but as clearing a plot of land to design a masterpiece. When the jaw is a room too small for all its inhabitants, creating space isn't just an option; it's the only way to let everyone breathe, to find their perfect place in the whole. When non-extraction methods are like trying to gently nudge people into place, extraction is the bold, necessary step of opening a new doorway.

The question then shifts from if we should make space, to how. And this is where the art begins.

The Classic Edit: The First Premolar Chapter

In the grand library of orthodontic tales, the most classic chapter involves the four first premolars. Positioned just behind the expressive canines—the cornerstones of the smile—these teeth hold a unique power. Removing them is the quintessential move, the "workhorse" that has shaped millions of confident smiles.

Why these four? Because their removal gifts the orthodontist with a precious currency: space. About 7-8 millimeters on both the upper and lower arches, to be exact. This isn't just a number; it's a breath of fresh air. It's the room needed to unravel a severe tangle of crowded teeth, allowing them to finally settle into a graceful, sweeping curve.

But their real magic lies in their ability to reshape a profile. When front teeth protrude, pushing the lips forward into a strained posture, the space created by removing the first premolars becomes a runway. It allows the orthodontist to gently guide those front teeth back, letting the lips fall into a soft, natural repose. It's a transformation that goes beyond the mouth; it redraws the silhouette of the face, bringing the entire facial structure into a quiet, confident balance. It's the difference between a story that feels forced and one that flows with effortless grace.

The Subtle Twist: The Second Premolar Gambit

But not every story calls for a dramatic edit. Sometimes, the narrative requires a more subtle touch, a strategic nuance that only a master storyteller would recognize. This is the domain of the second premolar extraction.

Choosing to remove the teeth just behind the first premolars is a move of quiet brilliance. It's for the patient whose facial profile is already beautifully balanced, where a significant pullback of the front teeth would be too much, potentially creating a "dished-in" or hollowed look. It's for when the crowding is more of a backstage issue, a traffic jam in the rear of the arch rather than a jumble at the front.

This choice is a masterclass in what orthodontists call "anchorage"—the art of a controlled tug-of-war. By removing the second premolars, the powerful first molars are left standing right next to the newly opened space. They become the unmovable anchors, the strongmen who hold the line, ensuring that the back teeth don't drift forward while the front teeth are gently nudged into place. Or, if the story requires it, these molars can be intentionally guided forward to close space and perfect the bite. It's a delicate dance of forces, a testament to the idea that the most powerful changes are often the most precise.

The Unconventional Narratives: Beyond the Premolars

Of course, the world of smiles is infinitely varied, and so are the solutions. While premolars are the main characters in most extraction stories, sometimes the plot demands a more unconventional hero.

Occasionally, the script calls for removing teeth only from the top arch, or only from the bottom. This is done to correct a mismatched relationship between the jaws, like a conversation where one speaker is leaning too far forward. By editing only one arch, the orthodontist can bring both into a harmonious dialogue.

In the rarest of tales, an incisor or a molar might be chosen for removal. This is never a first choice. It's a decision made only when a tooth is compromised by trauma or decay, or when the dental puzzle is so complex that this single, radical move is the key that unlocks the entire solution. These are the bold, bespoke strategies for truly unique cases, reminding us that every smile has its own journey.

The Digital Muse: Where Art Meets Algorithm

For generations, this intricate decision-making process was purely an art form, a wisdom held in the hands and eyes of the clinician. It was a craft honed over a lifetime of experience, a deep, intuitive understanding of facial harmony. But today, the artist has a powerful new partner: artificial intelligence.

AI is not here to write the story itself, but to serve as a brilliant analytical muse. Imagine an architect having a tool that could not only analyze the structural integrity of a building but also show a stunningly realistic projection of how the sunlight will fall through its windows at different times of day. That is what AI offers orthodontics.

By sifting through tens of thousands of successfully completed cases, AI models can now analyze a new patient's unique facial structure, bite, and crowding, and suggest the most promising extraction pattern with astonishing accuracy—some up to 86%. It can generate simulations, offering a glimpse into the future. Before a single bracket is placed, the orthodontist and the patient can sit together and see the potential final act: how the profile softens with first premolar extractions versus how it's subtly maintained with second premolar extractions.

This transforms the conversation. It replaces the leap of faith with a data-informed flight plan. It turns a complex, clinical choice into a collaborative, visual journey. The "guesswork" of the past is dissolving, replaced by an optimized path, a dialogue backed by probabilities and predictions.

The Unmistakable Human Touch

Yet, for all its power, AI is still just a tool. It is a compass, not the captain. The final decision will always, and must always, rest in the heart and mind of the human clinician.

The orthodontist is the one who sees beyond the data points. They understand the patient's anxieties, their hopes for their new smile, and the subtle nuances of their personality. They blend the cold, hard data from the AI with the warm, empathetic understanding of the person in their chair. They interpret the digital suggestions through the lens of lived experience, making the final, nuanced choice that feels right not just for the teeth, but for the human being they belong to.

The future of creating a smile is this beautiful fusion—where the timeless art of the human touch is elevated by the incredible precision of science. It's a partnership that ensures every story told by a smile is not only healthy and functional, but profoundly, uniquely, and beautifully its own.

Management of the Mixed Dentition: Interception and Guidance

The Guardians of the Smile: Why Tiny Teeth Hold the Key to a Healthy Future

For every parent, a child's bright, gap-toothed grin is a universe of joy. But behind that adorable smile, a carefully orchestrated symphony of growth is taking place. Those tiny baby teeth, often dismissed as mere "practice teeth," are in fact the unsung heroes of a healthy, beautifully aligned smile. They are the architects of the future, and when one is lost too soon, the entire blueprint can be thrown into disarray. This is where the magic of pediatric dentistry steps in, not just to fix problems, but to prevent them from ever happening.

The Domino Effect of a Single Lost Tooth

Imagine a perfectly set row of dominoes. Each one has its place, holding the potential for a flawless cascade. A child's primary teeth are much the same. They do more than just help your little one munch on apples and master their first words; they are the dedicated guardians of space, holding the exact spot for the permanent teeth that are patiently waiting their turn beneath the gums.

But what happens when one of these tiny guardians falls before its time? Whether due to a cavity that got a little too ambitious or an unexpected tumble on the playground, the premature loss of a baby tooth can trigger a silent, slow-motion chain reaction. The neighboring teeth, no longer feeling the gentle pressure of their companion, can begin to drift, like boats coming untethered from their moorings. The powerful permanent molar behind the gap might lean in, encroaching on the precious real estate.

This subtle shifting can create a roadblock for the incoming permanent tooth. When it's finally ready to make its grand entrance, it may find its path blocked, leading to a smile that's crowded, crooked, or worse, a tooth that becomes impacted, trapped beneath the surface with nowhere to go. This is the story of how small problems can grow into big ones, and it's why "space management" isn't just a dental term—it's a parent's superpower.

Meet the Space Maintainer: The Tiny Hero of the Gappy Grin

When a primary tooth is lost too soon, a pediatric dentist can call in a special hero: the space maintainer. Think of it as a custom-made placeholder, a tiny, silent guardian that steps in to hold the fort. It's a purely preventative measure, a way of pressing pause on the drifting of teeth, ensuring that when the new tooth is ready, its spot is waiting, open and welcoming.

These little marvels of dental engineering come in a few different forms, each tailored to the child's specific needs:

The Band and Loop: The most common type, this is like a tiny, custom-fit ring for a neighboring tooth with a delicate wire loop that extends across the gap, gently nudging the other tooth and saying, "This spot is taken!" It's a simple, elegant solution for the loss of a single molar.

The Lower Lingual Holding Arch (LLHA): When multiple baby teeth are lost on the lower jaw, a more robust hero is needed. The LLHA uses bands on the permanent molars and a discreet wire that runs along the inside of the lower front teeth. This acts as a sturdy barrier, preventing the back teeth from marching forward and the front teeth from tilting back.

The Nance Palatal Arch: The upper jaw's equivalent of the LLHA, this appliance uses a wire that sweeps across the roof of the mouth, often with a small acrylic button that rests against the palate. It's a silent sentinel, ensuring the upper molars stay put.

The Distal Shoe: This specialized appliance is for a very specific scenario: when a baby molar is lost before the first permanent molar has even arrived. A small part of the Distal Shoe actually extends beneath the gumline to guide the erupting permanent molar into its rightful place, like a gentle hand showing it the way.

When the Space Has Already Been Lost: Enter the Space Regainer

Sometimes, life gets in the way, and a child doesn't see a dentist right after a tooth is lost. In these cases, the neighboring teeth may have already started their migration, and a simple space maintainer won't be enough. This is when a space regainer is called into action.

If a space maintainer is a placeholder, a space regainer is an active mover. It's an orthodontic appliance that gently but persistently nudges the drifted teeth back into their original positions, reopening the space that was lost. Using tiny, calibrated springs or screws, a space regainer is a testament to the fact that even when things have gone a little off course, it's often possible to turn back the clock.

The Bigger Picture: An Investment in a Lifetime of Smiles

The conversation around space maintainers and regainers is about so much more than just teeth. It's about a philosophy of proactive, compassionate care that is at the heart of pediatric dentistry and orthodontics, a philosophy championed by leading institutions like Columbia and the University of Pennsylvania. It's about understanding that early, thoughtful intervention can prevent a cascade of issues down the road:

Avoiding Extensive Orthodontics: By preserving space, these simple appliances can dramatically reduce the need for more complex and costly orthodontic treatments in the teenage years.

Protecting Oral Health: A well-aligned smile is easier to clean, which means a lower risk of cavities and gum disease throughout a person's life.

Ensuring Proper Function: A healthy bite is crucial for everything from comfortable chewing to clear speech and even the healthy development of the jaw.

Nurturing Confidence: A beautiful, healthy smile is a source of confidence that can last a lifetime.

By embracing the power of space management, parents can become the ultimate guardians of their child's smile. It's a journey that transforms a simple dental visit into a powerful act of love, ensuring that the natural, beautiful plan for their child's smile can unfold, unhindered and full of promise.

A Smile's Architect: The Rare Art of Serial Extraction

In the story of your child's smile, each tooth is a character waiting to make its entrance. But what happens when the stage—the jaw itself—is simply too small for the entire cast? This is the heart of a common orthodontic challenge: a profound mismatch between the size of the permanent teeth and the arc of the jawbone destined to hold them. The result is severe crowding, a dental traffic jam that can compromise health, function, and the beautiful confidence we wish for every child.

In these specific and rare circumstances, orthodontics offers a path less traveled, a solution that requires foresight, courage, and incredible precision. It's called serial extraction.

This isn't about simply removing teeth. Think of it less as demolition and more as architectural planning for the mouth. Serial extraction is a carefully choreographed sequence of removing select primary (baby) teeth and, later, specific permanent teeth. The goal is not to create emptiness, but to grant freedom. It's about creating just enough space at just the right time, allowing the most important permanent teeth to glide into their natural, intended places, guided by nature's own eruptive forces. It's the art of making way for a masterpiece.

The Blueprint for a Balanced Smile: A Phased Journey

The classic serial extraction plan is a masterclass in timing, unfolding in harmony with a child's own developmental rhythm. It's a journey with three key phases, each designed to solve a problem before it becomes a crisis.

Phase 1: Creating Breathing Room for the Front

This first step typically happens around age 8 or 9, just as the permanent front teeth (the incisors) are making their debut. In a crowded jaw, this entrance is often chaotic—teeth emerge twisted, overlapped, or pushed out of line. By removing the primary canines (the small, pointed baby teeth), we perform an act of "unraveling." This simple procedure gives the incisors immediate relief and the space they need to align themselves naturally. It's like opening a window in a stuffy room, letting the fresh air—and the teeth—circulate into a healthier position.

Phase 2: Paving the Way for the Middle Act

About a year later, the focus shifts. The next set of characters, the permanent first premolars, are developing beneath the gums, waiting for their cue. To ensure their path is clear, the primary first molars are removed. This isn't just about making space; it's about accelerating a natural process. By removing the baby tooth, we encourage the permanent premolar to erupt sooner and more accurately, setting the stage perfectly for the final, most critical phase.

Phase 3: The Keystone Placement

This is the definitive step, usually performed between ages 10 and 12, when the newly erupted permanent first premolars are removed. Why remove a healthy, brand-new tooth? Because this strategic sacrifice creates the vital space needed for the true stars of the arch: the permanent canines. These "eyeteeth" are the cornerstones of a beautiful smile and a functional bite. Without this final intervention, they risk becoming impacted (stuck in the jawbone), erupting high on the gums, or forcing the other teeth into disarray. This last extraction ensures the canines have a clear, welcoming path to settle into the arch, locking the smile into a stable and harmonious state.

This entire blueprint is an act of interception. It's a commitment to addressing a severe issue early, with the hope of simplifying future treatment and giving the child a healthier, more stable foundation for life.

The Crossroads: Is This Journey Right for Your Child?

Embarking on the path of serial extraction is a profound decision, one made only after a meticulous diagnostic process. It is a solution for a very specific problem, not a universal fix. Here are the questions we must answer together to know if this is the right road:

Is the crowding truly severe? We're not talking about minor twists. This path is reserved for cases where there is a dramatic lack of space—a discrepancy of 7-10 millimeters or more. We use precise 3D scans, X-rays, and models to know the exact numbers.

Is the foundation solid? Serial extraction works wonders when the jaws themselves are in a healthy, balanced relationship (a Class I malocclusion). If the core issue is a skeletal imbalance—like a significantly recessed lower jaw or protrusive upper jaw—removing teeth can actually harm the facial profile.

Is the facial profile already pleasing? The goal is to preserve and enhance a child's natural beauty. For a child with a balanced profile, aligning the teeth can complete the picture. If extractions are done in the wrong case, they can lead to a flattened or "dished-in" look.

Are we solving a dental problem, not a skeletal one? This is the most important question. Serial extraction is a dental solution. Skeletal problems require different tools, sometimes including orthognathic surgery in combination with orthodontics.

Conversely, there are clear signs that this path is not the one to take. We would not consider serial extraction for mild or moderate crowding, for children who are naturally missing other permanent teeth, or for those with significant gaps or complex bite problems like an open bite. It requires a long-term commitment and unwavering cooperation from the patient and family.

The Modern Artisan and the Evolving Toolbox

In the world of modern orthodontics, the philosophy has shifted. The days of serial extraction as a common procedure are behind us. Why? Because the orthodontist's toolbox is fuller and more sophisticated than ever before.

Advanced 3D imaging allows us to predict growth with uncanny accuracy. Tools like palatal expanders can help us strategically widen the jaw itself, "creating" space that we once thought was impossible to gain. Modern braces and clear aligners are marvels of engineering, able to achieve complex movements with greater efficiency and comfort. The trend is rightly toward non-extraction therapies whenever possible, preserving every precious tooth.

Yet, serial extraction has not vanished. It has simply been refined. It remains an essential and powerful option for that small, specific group of children with severe, non-skeletal crowding.

Today, a modern serial extraction protocol is a bespoke plan, characterized by:

Pinpoint Diagnosis: Identifying the perfect candidate early in their development.

Meticulous Planning: Using digital tools to map out every step of the journey.

Patient Partnership: Ensuring the family is an educated and empowered member of the treatment team.

Integrated Finishing: Understanding that after the extractions have guided the teeth into place, a short phase of braces or aligners is often the final touch needed to perfect the alignment and close any remaining small spaces.

The Human Element: A Leap of Faith, A Lifetime Reward

Choosing serial extraction is an irreversible decision, and it's natural to feel apprehensive. It's a journey that can span several years, requiring patience and trust. When misdiagnosed, the side effects are significant—a compromised facial profile or spaces that are difficult to close.

But when it is the right answer, the benefits are life-changing. It allows teeth to move into place using their own natural energy, a more physiologic and stable process. It can dramatically shorten the time a child spends in full braces and, most importantly, it can rescue a smile from a future of severe crowding, impaction, and potential gum and bone damage.

Ultimately, serial extraction is a testament to the art and science of orthodontics. It's about looking at a crowded canvas and seeing the potential for a masterpiece. It's about having the wisdom to know when to intervene and the courage to make a bold move that will guide a child's developing smile toward a future of health, beauty, and confidence.

The Whisper of a Smile: A New Story in Children's Orthodontics

For generations, the path to a straight smile was a noisy one. It was a story told in metal, a journey marked by the click and clank of bulky expanders and the glint of partial braces. We called it Phase I, or "interceptive care," a clinical term for an often-uncomfortable reality for our children. The goal was noble: to guide growing jaws and make room for smiles to blossom. Yet, the tools we used, while effective, were a heavy burden for little shoulders. They could make a soft-spoken child quieter, a joyful eater hesitant, and a bright smile hide behind a self-conscious hand. It was a journey that often felt like a detour, a necessary hardship on the road to confidence.

But listen closely. Can you hear it? A quiet revolution is happening. A paradigm shift in orthodontics that speaks not in metal, but in a whisper. Today, we are rewriting the story of early treatment, trading the hardware of yesterday for the elegance of clear aligner therapy. This isn't just a new tool; it's a new philosophy, one that places a child's experience, their comfort, and their confidence at the very heart of the journey. We've moved from an era of interruption to one of gentle guidance, and in doing so, we're discovering we can nurture a child's growth in ways we once only dreamed of.

From Metal Mouths to Invisible Maps: The Evolution of a Child's Journey

Think back to the classic tale of early orthodontics. It was a story of correction, of intervening between the ages of 6 and 10 to tackle significant crowding or jaw misalignments before they set in stone. The heroes of this tale were cemented expanders and fixed-in-place braces—powerful, yes, but also demanding. They could turn a simple slice of pizza into a challenge and make the bristles of a toothbrush navigate an intricate maze. For a child navigating the delicate social world of the playground, the visible machinery in their mouth could feel like a spotlight, casting shadows on their self-esteem during their most formative years.

Then came the plot twist. The arrival of clear aligners for children was a pivotal moment, like switching from a loud, static-filled radio to crystal-clear surround sound. These are not just smaller versions of adult aligners; they are brilliant, custom-crafted maps for a growing smile. Imagine a series of virtually invisible, smooth plastic trays that are completely removable. This simple difference changes everything. The aesthetic advantage is profound—kids can laugh, talk, and learn without the social anxiety of traditional braces. But the magic goes deeper. Oral hygiene becomes simple again; they can brush and floss the teeth they were born with, not a complex appliance. The fear of breaking a bracket on a crunchy apple disappears, as aligners are removed for every meal, letting kids be kids.

Smart Smiles: Technology That Breathes with Your Child

This new chapter is powered by incredible technology designed with the dynamic, ever-changing world of a child's mouth in mind. One of the most inspired innovations is what we call "eruption compensation." Think of it as leaving a light on for a guest who has yet to arrive. Within the aligner trays, we create tiny, pre-planned spaces, like little bubbles, waiting patiently for permanent teeth to emerge. As a new tooth begins its ascent, the aligner doesn't block its path; it welcomes it, guiding it gently into its rightful place. It's a seamless dance between technology and nature, ensuring treatment works with a child's growth, not against it.

The process itself feels like something out of science fiction. We begin with a simple, comfortable 3D scan of your child's mouth, creating a stunningly precise digital blueprint. From there, we as orthodontists become choreographers, mapping out every subtle shift and movement from the first aligner to the final, radiant smile. This digital foresight gives us an unprecedented level of control. We can even include "compliance indicators"—tiny, colorful dots that fade with wear, acting as a secret handshake between parent, child, and orthodontist, ensuring the journey stays on track.

Unlocking Potential: What a Whisper Can Achieve

This gentler approach is remarkably powerful, capable of addressing the very same issues as its metallic predecessors, but with a grace and comfort that redefines the experience.

Widening a Smile, Finding Harmony: For a child with a narrow upper arch or a crossbite—where upper teeth tuck inside the lower ones—aligners can act like a gentle, steady guide. They progressively broaden the arch, creating the space needed for a full, healthy smile and correcting the bite. This early correction is vital, helping to prevent a lifetime of uneven tooth wear or jaw strain.

Balancing the Bite: In cases of a deep bite, where the top teeth hide the bottom ones, aligners can restore balance. Using tiny, strategically placed "bite ramps," they can gently reposition teeth to create a healthier, more comfortable and functional bite, protecting teeth from excessive wear and easing strain on the jaw joints.

The Guardians of Space: Perhaps the most proactive role aligners play is as guardians of the future smile. When a baby tooth is lost too soon, aligners can hold that precious space open, ensuring the permanent tooth has a clear path to erupt. They can prevent teeth from getting stuck or "impacted" and elegantly resolve crowding, setting the stage for a healthier dental future.

The New Conversation: When is it Time to Begin?

With this revolutionary tool in our hands, the conversation between parents and orthodontists has become richer and more nuanced. We're no longer just weighing the clinical pros and cons; we're considering the whole child.

The risk of "patient burnout"—of a child simply growing weary of a long, uncomfortable treatment—has always been a real concern. The financial and emotional investment of a two-phase treatment is significant. But because clear aligners dramatically reduce the daily burden on a child, the "cost" in terms of their happiness and cooperation is so much lower. This has lowered the threshold for when we might choose to intervene. A developing issue that we might have "watched and waited" on in the past can now be addressed proactively and gently, preventing it from becoming a bigger problem down the road.

This brings us to a fascinating concept: epigenetics. This is the idea that our environment and experiences can influence how our genes express themselves. In orthodontics, this is powerfully relevant. A child who breathes through their mouth due to allergies, for example, is environmentally predisposed to developing a narrow jaw and crooked teeth. Their genetics didn't doom them to this outcome; their environment shaped it. With the ease of clear aligners, we can now intervene earlier to counteract these environmental influences, guiding their growth back toward its healthier, natural potential.

Ultimately, the shift to clear aligners is fostering a more preventative and holistic philosophy. We are moving away from waiting for problems to become severe and towards a future where we can nurture growth from the very beginning. It's a quieter, kinder, and more collaborative approach—a partnership with parents and children to not just fix a smile, but to allow each child's unique, brilliant smile to truly flourish.

The Architect of the Smile: Unlocking Your Child's Potential

A child's smile is a masterpiece in the making. It holds the promise of future laughter, confidence, and connection. But sometimes, the foundation for that masterpiece—the upper jaw—is a little too narrow, creating a blueprint for future problems like crooked teeth and bite issues. For generations, the solution often involved waiting for problems to worsen, leading to more complex treatments later.

Today, we have a more enlightened approach. We can become the architects of our children's smiles, working with their natural growth to build a healthier, more harmonious foundation. This is the art and science of orthopedic expansion, a proactive journey that doesn't just straighten teeth, but reshapes the very canvas on which that future smile will be painted.

The Secret Seam: A Hidden Marvel of Childhood Growth

To understand this marvel, you have to know a secret about a child's upper jaw, the maxilla. It isn't one solid piece of bone. Instead, like two continents slowly drifting into place, its two halves are joined by a soft, flexible seam right down the center: the mid-palatal suture. This suture is a powerhouse of growth, a living line of cartilage designed by nature to widen as your child grows.

This pliable seam is the key. It's a window of opportunity unique to childhood. When genetics or habits cause the upper jaw to grow too narrow, we don't have to accept it. We can partner with the body's own growth engine, giving it a gentle, guiding nudge to fulfill its original, expansive blueprint. This is true architectural work—widening the very bone, not just tipping the teeth.

The Key to a Wider World: The Rapid Palatal Expander (RPE)

Our primary architectural tool is a remarkable device called the Rapid Palatal Expander (RPE). Custom-crafted for your child, this appliance is a silent partner in their growth. It fits snugly against the roof of the mouth, held in place by bands on the back teeth. At its heart is a small, powerful screw—think of it as the master key to unlocking the jaw's potential.

Whether it's the sleek, all-metal Hyrax design or a model that uses gentle acrylic pads to hug the palate, the RPE has one profound purpose: to deliver a slow, steady whisper of pressure across that central seam.

The Magic of Making Space

Here's where the magic happens. As a parent, you'll be given a special key to activate the expander. Once a day, with a simple, tiny turn, you become an active participant in this transformation. That turn sends a gentle signal across the suture, nudging the two halves of the maxilla apart by a fraction of a millimeter.

This isn't a forceful break, but a beautiful biological conversation. The suture responds by gradually separating. Soon, you might see a small gap appear between your child's two front teeth. Celebrate this gap! It's the definitive sign that you're not just moving teeth—you are creating new bone. You are making room for greatness.

The body, in its infinite wisdom, abhors a vacuum. It immediately dispatches its master builders—specialized cells called osteoblasts—to the site. They get to work, weaving new, healthy bone into the space that's been created. Day by day, turn by turn, you are helping to build a wider, stronger, and more spacious foundation for your child's smile.

The Blueprint for a Lifetime of Benefits

This architectural work has profound and lasting benefits, creating a cascade of positive changes.

A Balanced Foundation (Correcting Crossbites): Many children with narrow jaws have a posterior crossbite, where the top teeth bite uncomfortably inside the bottom teeth. This can force the jaw to shift to one side, leading to uneven wear, jaw joint strain, and even facial asymmetry. By widening the maxilla, the RPE corrects the foundation itself, allowing the bite to close in perfect, harmonious alignment.

An Open Floor Plan (Creating Space for Teeth): Think of the dental arch like the curved footprint of a house. By widening that footprint, we dramatically increase the available living space. This new real estate is priceless, creating the room needed for all the permanent teeth to emerge into their natural, beautiful positions without fighting for space.

Designing a Fuller, Healthier Smile (Avoiding Extractions): Perhaps the most celebrated benefit is that this process often makes the extraction of healthy permanent teeth completely unnecessary. Instead of removing teeth to solve a crowding problem, we solve the problem at its root by creating a jaw that is perfectly sized to house all of them. It's a philosophy of preservation, of honoring the body's original design.

The Finishing Touches: Patience and Partnership

Once the daily turns have achieved the perfect width, the most active part of your job is done. But the RPE's work isn't over. It now enters a quiet, crucial phase of "retention." For the next several months, the expander will remain in place, acting as a brace to hold the new, wider shape. This gives the body's construction crew the time it needs to fully mature and solidify the new bone, ensuring the beautiful foundation you've built will last a lifetime.

Being an architect of your child's smile is a partnership. It requires your commitment to those daily turns and your encouragement as your child adjusts to the new appliance. But this early, proactive step is one of the greatest gifts you can give them. By guiding their natural growth, you can simplify future treatments, improve the stability of their bite, and build a foundation for a lifetime of confident, radiant smiles. You're not just fixing a problem; you're unlocking the masterpiece that was there all along.

Contemporary Functional Appliances and Dentofacial Orthopedics for Class II Correction

The Face in Bloom: A Gardener's Guide to Growth

Imagine your child's growing face is like a rare and precious plant. For centuries, we believed its final form—the strong line of the jaw, the gentle curve of the profile—was completely decided by the genetic seeds from which it sprouted. We thought we could only stand back and watch it grow, for better or worse.

But what if we were wrong? What if we aren't just spectators, but gardeners?

This is the revolutionary promise of dentofacial orthopedics. It's a field built on a profound and beautiful idea: we can work with the body's natural intelligence, using gentle guidance to help the face bloom into its most harmonious and healthy form. This isn't about forcing nature, but partnering with it.

The Gardener's Secret: Listening to the Landscape

The secret lies in a groundbreaking concept called the functional matrix theory. Forget the old idea that bones are stubborn, pre-programmed architects of our face. Dr. Melvin Moss, the visionary behind the theory, proposed something far more elegant: bones are responsive followers. They are the trellis, and the surrounding life is the vine that shapes it.

Think about it. The powerful muscles you chew with, the tongue that forms words, the very space inside your mouth needed to breathe—these are the "functional tissues." They are the living, dynamic forces. Your jawbone doesn't just grow on its own; it listens. It grows and remodels itself in direct response to the needs and whispers of this bustling environment. If the muscles work differently, or the tongue needs more room, the bone dutifully reshapes itself to accommodate them.

This changes everything. If bone is an adapter, then it can be guided. We don't have to accept a blueprint; we can help draw a new one.

The Tools of Guidance: The Living Trellis

This is where functional appliances come in. These remarkable devices are not the brute force of traditional braces, which focus on pushing teeth into line. Think of a functional appliance as a living trellis, custom-built for the unique garden of your child's face.

These appliances—often removable, like a retainer—don't yank or pull. Instead, they change the environment. They gently encourage the lower jaw to sit in a new, healthier forward position. It's like placing a guide for a young vine. The appliance creates a new posture, a new set of tensions and spaces. It doesn't shout commands; it whispers a new suggestion to the body.

And the body, in its incredible wisdom, listens and responds.

A Symphony of Growth: Correcting a Receding Jaw

Let's watch this natural partnership in action, in one of the most common journeys: helping a lower jaw that hasn't grown as far forward as the upper jaw (a "Class II" profile).

The Gentle Invitation: The appliance holds the lower jaw forward, in a new, ideal relationship with the upper jaw. Immediately, the world changes for the facial muscles and tissues. They are stretched, like a dancer holding a new, elegant pose. This sustained new posture is a powerful signal sent deep into the body's growth centers.

Waking Up the Engine: The most magical part happens at the hinge of the jaw, near the ear. Here lies the condylar cartilage, a powerful engine of growth for the lower jaw. The new forward position, held by the appliance, acts like a key in the ignition. It stimulates the cells in this cartilage to multiply and create new bone. It's not just stretching; it's a genuine spark of new growth. The jawbone itself begins to grow longer, catching up to the upper jaw. This is true skeletal change, a fundamental rebalancing of the face from within.

The Whispering Brakes: At the same time, the gentle tension in the stretched cheeks and lips sends a different message to the upper jaw. This soft, constant pressure acts like a subtle brake, restraining the upper jaw's own forward growth. It's not about stopping it, but about coordinating a beautiful dance of growth between the two partners. By encouraging the lower jaw forward while reining in the upper, the entire facial profile moves toward harmony.

The Final Flourish: While the bones are reshaping, the teeth follow suit. The appliance helps guide the front teeth into a perfect bite, like arranging the final leaves and blossoms on the vine to perfectly catch the sun. These smaller movements are the finishing touch on the profound skeletal change happening beneath.

Of course, every gardener knows that success depends on a few key things. The patient must be a dedicated partner, wearing the "trellis" as prescribed to keep the gentle guidance constant. The timing must be right; this growth-guidance works best during the "growing season" of the pubertal growth spurt, when the body's potential is at its peak. And finally, it requires the eye of an expert orthodontist who understands not just mechanics, but the living, breathing biology of the individual.

Dentofacial orthopedics is more than a dental treatment. It's a dialogue with the body. It's a way to leverage the astonishing, adaptive nature of human life to cultivate not just a better bite, but a more balanced, confident, and harmonious face. It's the art of seeing the garden for the forest, and helping every feature find its place in the sun.

Imagine your jaw is a young dancer, a little shy, and not quite sure where to stand on the stage. It hangs back a bit, and as a result, the whole performance—your smile, your bite—is just a little off-key. For decades, orthodontists have had a clever set of choreographers for this exact problem: the first-generation functional appliances. Think of them as the classic dance instructors of the orthodontic world—the Twin Block, the Bionator, the Frankel. They're not about forcing a performance with rigid wires and brackets, but rather about teaching the dancer a new, more confident posture.

Take the Twin Block, for instance. It's less of an appliance and more of a dance partner. It consists of two smooth, separate plates for the upper and lower teeth, each with a small, angled ramp. When you close your mouth, these ramps meet and gently waltz your lower jaw forward into its ideal leading position. It's a subtle, persuasive cue, a constant reminder of where it needs to be. The magic isn't in brute force, but in this gentle, consistent guidance.

The Bionator acts more like a personal trainer, focusing on muscle memory. It encourages your tongue and jaw to adopt a healthier, forward-leaning posture, using your own muscle power to guide growth and alignment. The Frankel is different still; it's like an architect for your mouth. It uses shields to create space, holding back the powerful muscles of the cheeks and lips that can sometimes crowd the teeth. It essentially builds a bigger, more open "room" for your teeth to settle into, freeing them from restrictive pressures.

But here's the secret that underpins all of these brilliant designs: the dancer has to show up for practice. The magic of these appliances is unlocked only by the wearer. This is where the story shifts from the orthodontist's chair to the daily life of a teenager. For these appliances to work, they need to be worn, and not just for an hour or two. We're talking full-time commitment, a constant companion through homework, sleepovers, and binge-watching sessions, only taking a break for meals or sports. This is, and has always been, their greatest challenge and their most human element. Can you ask a teenager, already navigating the complex social currents of high school, to embrace this partner, this trainer, this architect, day in and day out?

Over the years, scientists and clinicians have put these classic choreographers to the test, moving beyond stories to hard evidence. What they've found is fascinating and nuanced. It turns out, a lot of the beautiful correction we see is more like clever stagecraft than a fundamental change in the dancer's anatomy.

Much of the improvement comes from what we call "dental tipping." Imagine the teeth are like furniture on the stage of your jaw. These appliances are masterful at rearranging that furniture. They can gently tilt the upper front teeth back and the lower front teeth forward, creating the perfect illusion of a perfectly aligned jaw. The bite looks and feels dramatically better, and for many, this is a fantastic result. It's a powerful and effective way to achieve a healthy smile.

What about actual jaw growth? Does the dancer's bone structure truly change? The evidence suggests that while these appliances can give growth a little nudge, the effect is modest. They don't typically produce the kind of dramatic, transformative jaw growth one might imagine. It's less like stretching the dancer's limbs and more like helping them stand up to their full, natural height during a crucial growth spurt. The science is clear: we can't create bone out of thin air, but we can absolutely work with the growth that nature provides.

This is why that human element—compliance—is the entire story. If the appliance is only worn sporadically, it's like a dance instructor who only shows up for half the lessons. The jaw never quite learns the new steps. The consistent, gentle pressure is what allows for both the beautiful dental rearrangements and the subtle encouragement of growth.

So, where does this leave our classic functional appliances? Not as outdated relics, but as trusted tools with a very specific, and still very relevant, purpose. They are not magic wands for creating new jaws, but they are brilliant at guiding teeth, improving bites, and working in harmony with a patient's natural development.

The journey with one of these appliances is a true partnership. It's a pact between the orthodontist, who understands the appliance's potential and its limits, and the patient, who holds the key to unlocking it. It's about setting realistic expectations—celebrating the artful rearrangement of teeth while appreciating the subtle influence on growth. The success story isn't written by the appliance itself, but by the dedicated young person who commits to the dance, day in and day out, guiding their own smile into its most confident and beautiful performance.

Taming the Stubborn Bite: A Guide to the Unsung Heroes of Orthodontics

Let's be honest. For decades, orthodontics has had a secret battle of wills. It's a silent struggle fought in households everywhere, centered around a simple question: "Are you wearing your retainer?" When it comes to fixing a significant overbite—what we call a "Class II malocclusion," where the lower jaw seems to be playing shy behind the upper jaw—this battle can feel like the main event. Traditional removable appliances are powerful tools, but they have an Achilles' heel: they only work if you wear them. And when they're left in their case, progress grinds to a halt.

But what if we could take that struggle completely off the table? What if we could enlist a silent partner in the journey to a perfect smile, one that works tirelessly, 24/7, without ever needing a reminder?

Enter the game-changers: fixed, non-compliance functional appliances.

Think of them as the special ops of orthodontics. These ingenious devices are cemented gently in place, becoming a seamless part of your mouth. They don't rely on memory or diligence; they rely on brilliant engineering. They are always on, always active, and always guiding the jaws toward their ideal harmony. While the legendary Herbst appliance is the well-known powerhouse of this family, clever specialists like the MARA and the Forsus Fatigue Resistant Device are also masters of their craft.

Now, these aren't magic wands. They are sophisticated tools that require a little extra care, like learning to navigate a new landscape in your mouth. They can make brushing a bit more of an adventure and are known for gently tipping the lower front teeth forward as part of their process. But understanding these unsung heroes—how they think, how they work, and how we manage their journey—is the key to unlocking their incredible power.

The Herbst: The Original Powerhouse

If fixed appliances were a team of superheroes, the Herbst would be the stoic, reliable leader. It's been on the scene for years, a true workhorse that has proven its mettle time and time again in the quest to correct overbites.

The Design: Imagine a tiny, custom-built hydraulic system for your jaw. The Herbst uses a brilliant pin-and-tube mechanism, like a miniature telescopic arm, that connects the back of the upper jaw to the front of the lower. This bridge doesn't lock you in place; it allows you to open and close comfortably, but it establishes a new "rule" for your lower jaw: you must close in a more forward, confident position. It essentially creates a new blueprint for how your bite comes together.

How it Works: The Herbst is a patient teacher, applying a constant, gentle nudge. This tireless persuasion accomplishes two amazing things:

A Growth Spurt on Demand: In a growing patient, this forward posture is like a personal trainer for the mandible, encouraging it to grow forward and catch up to the upper jaw.

A Gentle Rearrangement: It also strategically moves teeth, coaxing upper molars backward and lower molars forward, all to improve the fit. Of course, this forward pressure has a well-known sidekick effect: the lower front teeth tend to lean forward. This isn't a surprise; it's a predictable part of the journey that your orthodontist is already planning to address.

Living with the Herbst: Once the Herbst is placed, the "activation" is simply living your life. Your job is to become a master of hygiene, navigating the nooks and crannies with special brushes, and to be kind to the appliance by avoiding hard, sticky foods that could cause a breakdown. After about 6 to 12 months of this tireless work, the Herbst's job is done. It's removed to make way for the "finishing artists"—traditional braces that will perfect the details and upright those front teeth.

The MARA: The Sleek Minimalist

The Mandibular Anterior Repositioning Appliance (MARA) is the elegant, streamlined member of the team. It achieves the same incredible results as the Herbst but with a slightly less bulky profile.

The Design: Instead of telescopic rods, the MARA uses smooth, curved "elbows" attached to the molars. When you bite down, these elbows meet and guide the lower jaw smoothly into its new forward home. It's a simpler, more understated design that many patients find very comfortable.

How it Works: The philosophy is the same: constant, gentle guidance. The MARA is a quiet force for change, promoting jaw growth and shifting teeth into a healthier relationship. And yes, like its cousin the Herbst, it will encourage the lower incisors to tip forward as it works its magic—a temporary phase on the path to the final goal.

The Forsus: The Flexible Persuader

The Forsus Fatigue Resistant Device is the flexible, energetic specialist of the group. It's known for its incredibly light, continuous force that feels more like a gentle suggestion than a firm push.

The Design: The Forsus is essentially a tiny, sophisticated spring. It attaches to the braces on your upper molars and connects to the wire on your lower teeth. As you close, the spring compresses, delivering a continuous, gentle forward thrust to the lower jaw. Its flexible nature allows for a fantastic range of motion, making it feel surprisingly unobtrusive.

How it Works: The compressed spring is the engine of the Forsus, working around the clock to advance the lower jaw. It accomplishes the same trio of effects: encouraging jaw growth, shifting molars, and, you guessed it, causing some forward tipping of the lower front teeth. Some believe its flexible nature makes this tipping slightly less pronounced, but it's still a key factor your orthodontist will masterfully manage.

The Rules of the Road: Caring for Your Appliance

Whichever of these amazing appliances is chosen for your journey, the path to success has a few clear signposts:

Hygiene is Everything: This is non-negotiable. These appliances create new hiding spots for food and plaque. Becoming a brushing and flossing champion (perhaps with the help of a water flosser or interdental brushes) is your most important job. It protects your investment in your smile.

Respect the Hardware: Treat your appliance like the high-performance machine it is. A softer diet is your friend. Hard candies, sticky caramels, and crunchy nuts are its enemies. Avoiding them prevents emergency repair visits.

Embrace the Adjustment: The first few days will feel strange. Your cheeks and muscles need to get used to their new companion. This is normal. A little orthodontic wax and over-the-counter pain relievers can be your best friends during this short adjustment period.

Trust the Plan: Remember that these appliances are just Phase One. They do the heavy lifting of correcting the jaw relationship. Phase Two—almost always a period in traditional braces—is where the artistry happens. This is when your orthodontist will meticulously align every tooth, fine-tune your bite, and expertly correct any side effects, like tipping those lower incisors back into their perfect, upright position.

The Grand Finale

Fixed functional appliances are more than just metal and springs; they are a brilliant solution to a long-standing orthodontic puzzle. By taking the burden of compliance off the patient's shoulders, they clear the way for predictable, incredible, and life-changing results.

They represent a partnership between clever engineering and your body's natural potential. While they demand a little extra care and attention, the payoff is enormous: the taming of a stubborn bite and the creation of a healthy, beautiful smile that was always waiting to be revealed. They are the unsung heroes who work silently behind the scenes, ensuring that the final result is nothing short of spectacular.

The Ghost in the Smile: How an Old-School Gadget Still Teaches Us to Build a Face

There's a memory, a faint echo for many, of a classmate, a cousin, or maybe even yourself. It's a nighttime ritual, the quiet click of a strap, the cool metal frame tracing the curve of the cheeks. It's the orthodontic headgear, a device that feels more like a relic from a bygone era than a piece of modern medicine. For decades, this was the architect's heavy machinery in the world of orthodontics, the go-to tool for the toughest jobs in reshaping a smile.

Imagine an orthodontist not just as a tooth-straightener, but as a facial architect. Their job wasn't merely to arrange the furniture—the teeth—but to influence the very walls and foundations of the room: the jaws. Headgear was their crane and their scaffold. With a strap around the neck or head connected to a "facebow," it applied a gentle, persistent force that could achieve something remarkable. It could whisper to a young, growing upper jaw, "Slow down, you're growing too fast," correcting a significant overbite by addressing its skeletal source. It could nudge the big back molars rearward, like pushing back a wall to create more living space in a crowded room. It was the anchor, the unmovable force that held the line while other teeth were carefully guided into their rightful place. It wasn't just moving teeth; it was shaping growth, a true feat of biological engineering.

The Rise of the Interior Designers

Then, the world of orthodontics had its own quiet revolution. New tools arrived, sleek, subtle, and incredibly clever. Tiny titanium screws, called Temporary Anchorage Devices (TADs), could be placed directly into the bone inside the mouth, creating an invisible, immovable anchor point. At the same time, a new generation of "fixed functional" appliances came on the scene—intricate springs and hinges that worked inside the mouth to encourage the lower jaw to grow forward.

These new kids on the block were the interior designers of orthodontics. They were brilliant at working within the existing architecture. They were discreet, often completely hidden. Most importantly, they freed the patient from the burden of remembering to use them. They were always on, always working, a silent, tireless force. The appeal was undeniable. Patients and orthodontists began to favor these less visible, "non-compliant" solutions that didn't demand hours of dedicated wear. The age of the external scaffold seemed to be fading.

When You Still Need to Move a Wall

And yet, headgear never truly vanished. It retreated from the spotlight, its role becoming more specialized, but in its niche, it remains a tool of profound power. Why? Because sometimes, interior design isn't enough. Sometimes, you have to move a wall.

Headgear's unique, enduring value lies in its ability to perform that grand architectural feat: directly influencing the growth of the upper jaw bone. This "orthopedic" effect is something that internal appliances struggle to replicate in the same way. For a young, growing child whose upper jaw is significantly overgrown, headgear can still be the most direct, most biologically sound way to guide their facial development into balance. It can prevent the need for much more invasive jaw surgery down the road.

This is where the artistry of the orthodontist comes in, choosing the right tool for the job:

A Cervical-Pull Headgear, with its neck strap, acts like a gentle anchor pulling backward and slightly downward—perfect for guiding the jaw and helping to correct a deep bite.

A High-Pull Headgear, anchored from the top of the head, pulls backward and upward. This is the tool for rotating the facial blueprint, ideal for patients where controlling vertical growth is key.

The lesser-known cousin, the Reverse-Pull Headgear (or Facemask), does the opposite. For children with an underdeveloped upper jaw (an "underbite"), it braces against the chin and forehead to pull the entire upper jaw forward, a life-changing intervention for the right patient.

This is not just moving teeth. This is shaping a face.

The Human Factor: The Price of Power

The great trade-off, the dramatic tension in the story of headgear, has always been compliance. Its power is directly tied to the patient's willingness to wear it. An architectural blueprint is useless if the construction crew doesn't show up for work. Twelve to fourteen hours a day, every day. It's a huge ask, especially for a teenager navigating the social minefield of middle or high school.

The feeling of being "different," the nightly discipline, the faint pressure during sleep—this is the human cost of headgear's power. It's the reason why the "set it and forget it" appeal of modern, internal appliances is so strong. They remove the human variable of compliance from the equation, offering a more predictable path to success.

The Future is a Collaboration

Today, orthodontics is not about old versus new. It's about having a rich, diverse toolkit and the wisdom to know when to use each tool. The future may lie in combining these approaches. Perhaps a short, effective course of headgear during a critical growth spurt to handle the heavy skeletal lifting, followed by sleek aligners or internal devices to perfect the details.

We are entering an era of "smart" orthodontics, with sensors that could one day track wear-time and forces, giving the orthodontist a perfect picture of what's happening. But the core lesson of headgear remains. It reminds us that a beautiful smile is more than just straight teeth. It's the product of a balanced, healthy foundation. While it may no longer be the star of every show, the old architect of the face is still on call, ready for those profound cases where you don't just rearrange the furniture, you rebuild the room.

Advanced Strategies for Class III Correction in Growing Patients

Of all the stories a human face can tell, one of the most compelling is written in the smile. Sometimes, that story involves a unique harmony, a puzzle of sorts, where the lower jaw steps forward to greet the world a little more boldly than the upper. This is the landscape of a Class III malocclusion, often known as an underbite. But before an orthodontist can help cultivate a new, more balanced smile, they must first become a student of that person's unique story, understanding not just the "what," but the "why" and the "what's to come."

The Fork in the Road: A True Path or a Detour?

Imagine standing at a trail entrance. Two paths lead into the woods. One is a winding, challenging mountain trail, etched into the landscape itself. The other is a simple, flat path that has a fallen log blocking the way. From the entrance, they might look like they lead to the same difficult place, but the journey is profoundly different. This is the most critical choice in treating a Class III bite: distinguishing the mountain from the log.

The Detour: A "Pseudo" Class III

The path with the fallen log is what we call a "pseudo-Class III." Here, the landscape of the jaws—the actual bone structure—is fundamentally balanced and harmonious. The blueprint is perfect. However, a single tooth or a group of teeth may have emerged in just the wrong spot, creating a tiny, uncomfortable collision when the person tries to bite. To avoid that little bump in the road, the person unconsciously learns a detour. They guide their lower jaw forward into a new "comfort zone," which creates the illusion of an underbite.

The patient isn't built this way; they've adapted. The treatment, then, isn't about reshaping the mountains. It's simply about removing the log. With minor adjustments, the orthodontist clears the interference, and like a traveler finding the true path, the jaw can finally relax back into its natural, intended position. The journey is often short, simple, and transformative.

The Mountain Trail: A True Skeletal Class III

The mountain trail is a "true skeletal Class III." This isn't an adaptation; it's the landscape itself. The genetic blueprint has called for a lower jaw that is perhaps a bit more expressive and larger, or an upper jaw that is a touch more reserved and set back. It might be a combination of both. This is a structural reality, woven into the very bones of the face. You cannot simply ask the jaw to "go back," any more than you could ask a mountain to move. Understanding this is everything, because you don't treat a mountain the same way you treat a fallen log.

Reading the Landscape: The Art of Forecasting Growth

Once an orthodontist confirms they are looking at a true mountain trail, the next, and perhaps most profound, challenge begins: understanding the weather. A child's face is not a static photograph; it's a living, growing season. The central question becomes: how will this landscape change over time? Will the lower jaw's growth be a gentle, rolling hill, or will it be a dramatic, soaring peak? Predicting this growth is the art that informs the science of treatment.

This forecast determines the entire approach. For some, the growth pattern might be mild enough that the final skeletal imbalance can be "camouflaged." Think of it as clever landscaping—skilfully arranging the teeth so that even if the underlying foundation isn't perfectly level, the final garden is beautiful, functional, and harmonious.

For others, however, the growth pattern is a powerful, relentless force. Camouflage would be like planting flowers on the side of an active volcano—a temporary fix against an overwhelming natural power. For these individuals, the most stable, healthy, and beautiful result will ultimately involve waiting for the seasons of growth to complete, and then partnering with a surgeon to reshape the mountain itself through orthognathic (jaw) surgery.

The Tools of the Gardener-Architect

To read this living landscape and forecast its future, the orthodontist becomes part gardener, part architect, using specialized tools to see beyond the surface.

The Blueprint of the Skull (Cephalometric Radiographs): The "ceph" is the master blueprint. This special X-ray allows the orthodontist to see the precise architecture of the face and jaws. Angles and lines are drawn on this map to reveal the story of the bones.

The SNA angle tells of the upper jaw's place in the world. Is it prominent or shy?

The SNB angle speaks to the character of the lower jaw. Is it forward-thinking and assertive?

The ANB angle is the relationship between the two—the dialogue between the jaws. A negative ANB is the classic signature of a skeletal Class III landscape.

Other measurements, like the Wits Appraisal and Mandibular Plane Angle, add further chapters to the story, describing the jaw's position and the steepness of its climb.

Reading the Seasons of Growth: A single blueprint is just one moment in time. To truly understand the future, the orthodontist must read the seasons.

Cervical Vertebral Maturation (CVM): By observing the changing shapes of the neck vertebrae on the ceph, an orthodontist can see if the patient is in the springtime of their growth, the peak of their adolescent summer growth spurt, or entering the autumn of growth completion. This avoids extra radiation and provides a remarkably accurate growth calendar.

Hand-Wrist Radiographs: Similar to CVM, the bones in the hand mature in a predictable sequence, offering another window into the patient's personal season of growth.

Family History: Genes are the memory of the landscape. Looking at the smiles of parents and siblings offers powerful clues about the path a young person's growth may follow.

The Living Story: Most importantly, the orthodontist watches the story unfold in real-time. By comparing blueprints taken over months or years, they can see the exact pace and direction of change, turning a forecast into a direct observation.

This deep, multi-faceted diagnosis is the soul of treatment. It's what allows an orthodontist to recommend with confidence whether to intervene early with growth-guiding appliances, to wait and create a beautiful camouflage with braces, or to plan for a future surgical correction that will provide a lifetime of stability and confidence.

In the end, navigating a Class III malocclusion is a profound journey. It begins with the wisdom to distinguish a simple detour from a majestic mountain and continues with the art of reading the seasons of a growing human being. It's a partnership built on foresight, trust, and a shared goal: to cultivate a healthy, harmonious smile that tells a story of confidence for years to come.

The Smile's Blueprint: A Different Kind of Superhero Story

Every child's face holds a unique story, a blueprint for the person they are becoming. But sometimes, the architectural plans get a little out of sync. Imagine the upper and lower jaws are two partners in a dance who aren't quite in step. The lower jaw, bold and enthusiastic, steps a little too far forward, while the upper jaw, perhaps a bit shy, hangs back. This creates a disharmony—a bite that doesn't quite meet, known as a Class III relationship. Left to its own devices, this imbalance can shape not just a child's profile, but their confidence and comfort.

But what if we could give that shy upper jaw a gentle, guiding hand? What if we could nudge it forward, encouraging it to take its rightful place in the dance? This is the mission of the orthopedic facemask, a remarkable tool that isn't just about straightening teeth, but about reshaping the very foundations of a smile. It's less a medical device and more a piece of training gear for a young superhero on a quest to bring their own face into beautiful balance.

The Growth Guide: How to Wake a Sleeping Jaw

Forget intimidating metal contraptions. Think of the facemask as a personal growth guide. It's worn outside the mouth, featuring a soft cushion that rests on the forehead and a gentle cup that cradles the chin. These are the anchors, the steady base camp for the journey ahead. Connecting them is a light, vertical frame.

From this frame, tiny elastic bands—like super-strong, gentle bungee cords—reach into the mouth, connecting to a custom-fit appliance on the upper teeth. Once connected, a whisper-quiet conversation begins. The elastics deliver a continuous, soft nudge, a persistent "come-forward" signal to the upper jaw. This isn't a forceful pull; it's a persuasive invitation. The direction is precise: forward and slightly downward, a combination that helps "un-stick" the jaw from its recessed position and coax it into the light.

The real magic happens deep within the facial structure, at the growth seams, or sutures. In a growing child, these seams are like fertile ground, full of potential. They are not yet locked into place. The steady tension from the facemask acts like sunlight on a seedling, stimulating these areas to create new bone. It's the body's own incredible power of creation, awakened by a gentle, consistent request. At these seams—connecting the jaw to the cheekbones, the nose, and the very back of the skull—new growth blossoms, effectively lengthening the upper jaw and moving the entire mid-face forward. This isn't just about moving teeth; it's about guiding the growth of the very bone that holds them.

The Unveiling: A New Harmony in Form and Function

When a child partners with their facemask, the results can be transformative, revealing the balanced profile that was always waiting in their blueprint.

A Rewritten Profile: The most profound change is seeing the child's face come into harmony. The upper jaw moves forward, softening a prominent chin and filling out a "dished-in" mid-face. A profile that was once concave begins to straighten, blossoming into a balanced and aesthetically pleasing contour. This is the skeleton itself responding, creating a permanent, foundational shift that will support them for a lifetime.

A Smile That Clicks: While the bones are the main characters, the teeth play a crucial supporting role. As the upper jaw advances, the front teeth naturally follow, gliding into their correct position over the lower teeth. The bite, once misaligned, finally "clicks" into place. This achieves more than just a beautiful smile; it creates a functional, efficient bite for chewing and clearer speech.

The Ripple Effect of Confidence: The ultimate outcome is seen not just in X-rays and dental models, but in the child themselves. It's in the confident, easy smile, the boost in self-esteem, and the freedom from potential jaw surgeries down the road. It's the powerful gift of intercepting a problem early and setting a child on a healthier, more confident path.

The Quest's Companion: Realities of the Journey

Like any heroic quest, the journey with a facemask has its own set of challenges and truths. Understanding them is key to success.

The Secret Window of Time: This magic is only possible during a specific, fleeting chapter of childhood, typically between the ages of 7 and 10. This is the enchanted window when the facial seams are still open and responsive. As a child ages, these seams begin to fuse, and the window closes. Early detection is everything; it's the key that unlocks the possibility of this gentle, transformative treatment.

The Hero's Pact: The facemask's power is directly tied to the child's commitment. It requires a pact—a promise to wear the "training gear" for about 12 to 14 hours a day, mostly while sleeping and relaxing at home. This is where the real heroism lies. It takes dedication from the child and a universe of support from their family. It can feel awkward or cumbersome at first, but with encouragement and focus on the goal, it becomes a routine part of the quest. Consistent wear is the fuel for change.

The Unfinished Story: One of the greatest challenges is that our jaws grow on their own timetables. The lower jaw often continues its growth spurt into the late teens, long after the upper jaw has finished. This means that even after a perfect correction, a late surge of lower jaw growth can sometimes create a partial relapse. The story isn't always over when the facemask is put away. It simply means the quest may have a second chapter, perhaps with braces or retainers, to maintain the beautiful harmony that was achieved.

In the end, the orthopedic facemask is a testament to the incredible partnership between thoughtful science and the body's own potential for growth. It's a tool that empowers a child not just to change their bite, but to take an active role in shaping their own future, one gentle, forward nudge at a time.

The Unseen Architect: Reshaping a Smile from the Inside Out

Imagine a young person, maybe your own child, standing at the threshold of their teenage years. It's a time of navigating friendships, discovering passions, and figuring out who they are. But for some, this journey is overshadowed by a quiet struggle, one that's written on their very face. Their lower jaw might be growing with a little too much enthusiasm, or their upper jaw seems hesitant to keep pace. Doctors call it a "Class III malocclusion," but for a teen, it can feel like a spotlight on their biggest insecurity.

For years, the go-to solution was the facemask, a cumbersome external device worn for hours a day. It was a visible symbol of their treatment, a constant reminder of their difference. And its success rested heavily on their young shoulders, demanding a level of discipline that's tough for any kid juggling school, sports, and a social life. While a valiant effort, the facemask often felt like trying to steer a ship by pulling on its sails, when what you really need is to guide the rudder.

But what if we could work with the body's own blueprint? What if we could become unseen architects, working beneath the surface to guide the foundations of the face into harmony? This is the dawn of a new era in orthodontics, a beautifully orchestrated blend of surgical finesse and orthodontic vision. It's a technique known as Bone-Anchored Intermaxillary Traction, and at its heart are tiny, revolutionary tools called "Bollard plates." This isn't just about straightening teeth; it's about reshaping a future.

More Than Metal: The Tiny Anchors of Change

Forget what you know about traditional braces. Bollard plates are something else entirely. Picture small, exquisitely crafted titanium plates, no bigger than a pinky fingernail. Titanium is the chosen material not for its strength alone, but for its unique ability to whisper to the body in a language it understands. It's biocompatible, a welcome guest that the bone doesn't just tolerate, but embraces.

These aren't clunky pieces of hardware. They are discreet and elegant in their design, featuring a smooth plate that rests on the bone and a small, polished hook that peeks out, ready to do its work. Think of them not as implants, but as tiny, steadfast anchors dropped directly into the skeletal landscape of the jaw. This direct connection is their superpower, the secret to their profound and precise influence.

A Gentle Beginning: The Art of Placement

The journey begins not with the clinking of orthodontic wires, but with the quiet precision of a surgeon's hands. In a minor procedure, often performed with the patient comfortably sedated, an oral surgeon becomes a sculptor. Tiny incisions, carefully placed, reveal the bone of the upper and lower jaws.

With the skill of a watchmaker, the surgeon secures these Bollard plates to very specific, pre-planned locations – near the cheekbones on the upper jaw and behind the molars on the lower. This placement is a masterclass in collaboration, a map drawn by both the orthodontist and the surgeon to ensure the forces will be applied in the perfect direction. Once the plates are in place, the gums are gently nestled back around them, leaving only the small, unassuming hooks visible.

Then, nature performs its quiet miracle. Over the next few weeks, a process called "osseointegration" begins. It's a beautiful word for a beautiful phenomenon: the living bone cells reach out and literally fuse with the titanium plates, locking them into an unshakable embrace. The plates cease to be foreign objects and become a part of the patient's own body, a solid foundation from which to build a new smile.

The Invisible Engine: A Constant, Gentle Guidance

With the anchors secure, the orthodontist steps in to start the engine. This is where the magic of "traction" happens. Small, powerful elastics—like tiny, dedicated personal trainers—are stretched between the hooks on the upper and lower plates.

Imagine an invisible, internal force, a constant, gentle hum of energy working 24 hours a day. This force is pure and direct. It doesn't push and pull on the teeth, asking them to do the heavy lifting. Instead, it speaks directly to the bone. It's a whisper of encouragement to the upper jaw, coaxing it forward. It's a gentle hand on the shoulder of the lower jaw, guiding its growth.

The patient wears these elastics faithfully, a small, daily ritual that powers a profound transformation. They can eat, talk, and laugh without a bulky external appliance. The work is happening silently, powerfully, from the inside out.

Sculpting Bone, Not Just Shifting Teeth

This is what makes Bollard plates a true game-changer. The results are "purely orthopedic," meaning the change is happening at the skeletal level. The very foundation of the face is being reshaped.

A Blooming Upper Jaw: The maxilla is encouraged to grow to its full potential, creating better support for the mid-face.

A Harmonized Lower Jaw: The forward thrust of the mandible is gracefully controlled and redirected.

Happier, Healthier Teeth: By bypassing the teeth, we avoid the unwanted side effects of tipping or straining them, leading to a more stable, beautiful, and lasting result.

This approach is reserved for those who need it most—growing children and teens with significant jaw discrepancies. It's a powerful intervention that stands in the gap between traditional orthodontics and major jaw surgery. For many, it's the key that unlocks the possibility of avoiding complex surgery later in life. For others, it simplifies any future procedures, making them less invasive and more predictable.

The Journey to a New Horizon

Embarking on this treatment is a partnership. It requires a small act of bravery for the initial placement, followed by the quiet discipline of wearing elastics. But the patient is never alone. They are surrounded by a team—a surgeon, an orthodontist, and a supportive family—all working towards a single goal.

The transformation is often gradual, then suddenly apparent. It's in the way their profile softens. It's in the new confidence of their smile. It's the moment they realize they no longer hide their face in photos. Bollard plates represent more than just advanced medicine; they represent a deeper understanding of growth, a more compassionate approach to correction, and a hopeful pathway for young people to grow into the truest and most confident version of themselves. It is the art of shaping the future of a smile, one bone-anchored, life-changing step at a time.

The Underbite's New Groove: A Story of Jaws, Innovation, and Shifting the Bite

For as long as we've been straightening teeth, the underbite—known in clinical circles as a Class III malocclusion—has been one of the toughest puzzles to solve. It's a story written in the profile, where the lower jaw steps forward too boldly, or the upper jaw hangs back a bit shyly. For generations, the solutions felt like something out of a medieval playbook: bulky, cage-like headgear worn at night, or the daunting prospect of jaw surgery. The journey was often long, complex, and socially awkward.

But orthodontics is a story of relentless innovation, a quiet revolution happening inside the mouth. In recent years, a new character has entered the scene, a sleek, intraoral device promising a different, more elegant first act for Class III correction. It's called the Carriere Motion 3D Class III appliance, and it's part of a philosophy that's changing the entire rhythm of treatment.

The Diplomat of the Jaws

Imagine you have a complex negotiation between two opposing parties—in this case, your upper and lower jaws. Instead of launching into an all-out campaign with a full set of braces, you first send in a diplomat to broker a key agreement. That, in essence, is the Carriere appliance.

It's a small, smooth metal arm, discreetly bonded to two upper teeth—typically the canine and the first molar. From a tiny hook on this arm, a simple elastic band stretches down to an anchor point in the lower jaw. It's a fixed, yet surprisingly minimalist, setup. This is the heart of what its creators call the "Sagittal First Philosophy," a strategy that says: let's solve the main front-to-back problem first, before we deal with anything else.

The appliance acts like a trailblazer. As the patient wears the elastic, it delivers a steady, gentle, backward pull. The goal isn't just to tug on one or two teeth; it's to get the entire lower arch, from the back molar to the canine, to move backward as a single, harmonious unit. The Carriere aims to establish a peaceful "Class I" relationship—the dental equivalent of a perfect handshake—before the comprehensive treatment of braces or aligners even begins. By pre-correcting the bite, it promises to simplify everything that follows, potentially shaving months off the total treatment time.

The Great Debate: Rearranging the Furniture vs. Moving the Walls

So, how does this little diplomat work its magic? This is where we get to the most fascinating question in orthodontics: are we just moving teeth around, or are we actually changing the jaws themselves? Think of it like this: are we just rearranging the furniture in a room (a dental effect), or are we moving the walls of the house (a skeletal effect)?

The Carriere appliance is a master of interior design. For adults, its effects are overwhelmingly dental. It skillfully repositions the teeth, tipping and sliding them into a better alignment that brilliantly masks the underlying skeletal discrepancy. Profile improvements are often the result of this clever dental choreography, not a fundamental change in the jawbones.

For patients who are still growing, the story gets a little more nuanced. The hope is that the persistent force can act more like a gentle guide for the growing skeleton, perhaps discouraging the lower jaw's forward rush while nudging the upper jaw along. It's here that the appliance might dip its toes into the waters of skeletal change. However, the scientific community is still in a lively debate about how much of this is the appliance's influence and how much is just natural growth. The consensus for now? The Carriere is a phenomenal tooth-mover, and any skeletal changes are more of a subtle whisper than a shout.

Listening to the Evidence and the Human Factor

While glowing reports and clinical success stories abound, the broader scientific evidence paints a more measured picture. Many studies confirm that the Carriere is highly effective at what it promises: moving teeth to create that ideal "Class I platform." But these studies often come with footnotes. Many lack control groups, making it hard to isolate the appliance's work from the body's own developmental script.

And then there's the all-important human factor: the elastics. The Carriere's success is directly tethered to a patient's commitment to wearing those little rubber bands as instructed. Without that cooperation, the diplomat's mission fails. This highlights a universal truth in orthodontics: the most brilliant device is only as effective as the person wearing it.

The New Frontier: When Orthodontics Gets Superpowers

The Carriere's philosophy of simplifying treatment fits perfectly into a larger trend that is radically reshaping the field. Orthodontics is becoming bolder, seeking more predictable and powerful ways to tackle the toughest cases. This new frontier is being driven by the power of "skeletal anchorage."

If the Carriere is a diplomat, skeletal anchorage is like bringing in a team of structural engineers with superpowers. Using tiny, temporary titanium screws or plates (TADs) anchored directly into the jawbone, orthodontists can now apply forces with pinpoint precision and incredible control. These "bone anchors" provide an immovable foundation, allowing for movements that were once thought impossible without surgery.

With skeletal anchorage, orthodontists can:

Truly Move the Walls: In growing and even some adult patients, they can apply forces directly to the bone to encourage or redirect jaw growth, achieving genuine skeletal change.

Eliminate Side Effects: They can move entire sections of teeth without the reciprocal push-and-pull that can cause unwanted movement elsewhere.

Redefine "Impossible": They are successfully treating complex Class III cases in adults that, just a decade ago, would have been sent straight to a surgeon.

This is where the line between orthodontics and orthopedics blurs into an exciting new territory.

The Carriere Motion appliance holds its own unique and valuable place in this evolving story. It represents a brilliant strategy of efficiency—a way to elegantly set the stage for a simpler, faster finish. But it also reminds us that for the most profound changes, for those cases that require moving the very foundation of the smile, the future lies in harnessing the power of the bone itself. The journey to the perfect bite is no longer a single, prescribed path, but a rich landscape of innovative tools and philosophies, all working toward one beautiful goal: a healthy, functional, and confident smile.

Part III: Innovations in Treatment Modalities and Technology

The Fully Digital Orthodontic Workflow: From Scan to In-House Appliance Fabrication

The End of the Goop: Your Smile's Digital Debut

Let's be honest. If you could time-travel, you probably wouldn't set the dial for a dental appointment in the 1990s. Specifically, you'd want to leapfrog the moment that tray of cold, gooey, vaguely mint-flavored putty was aimed at your wide-open mouth.

Remember that feeling? The slow, creeping ooze, the gentle pressure that felt anything but, and the internal monologue screaming, Don't gag, don't gag, don't gag. For decades, this was the necessary evil of dentistry—the price of admission for a crown, a bridge, or braces. This messy, cumbersome ritual produced a plaster-of-paris model of your teeth, a chalky, fragile ghost of your smile that was the foundation for your entire treatment. It was a process that belonged more in a sculptor's dusty studio than in a modern healthcare setting.

But that era is over. The gateway to modern dentistry isn't a tray of goop; it's a slender, elegant wand that feels like it was designed by Apple. Welcome to the age of the intraoral scanner (IOS), the device that has single-handedly retired the gag-inducing impression tray to the museum of dental history.

A Storyteller for Your Smile

Imagine a device, no bigger than your electric toothbrush, gracefully dancing over your teeth. This is the intraoral scanner. It's not just taking pictures; it's a digital storyteller, capturing the epic saga of your smile in thousands of frames per second. Using a cascade of light, it meticulously maps every peak, valley, and subtle contour of your teeth and gums.

On a screen beside you, a universe materializes in real-time. A stunningly detailed, three-dimensional digital twin of your mouth is born. You can spin it, zoom in, and see your own smile from angles you never thought possible. It's not a static, lifeless cast; it's a dynamic, interactive blueprint, a living map of your oral world. This isn't just an improvement; it's a revolution in comfort and understanding. The awkward, messy ordeal of the past has been replaced by a quick, fascinating, and utterly comfortable digital light show.

Beyond a Pretty Picture: The Digital Difference

The magic of the intraoral scanner isn't just in avoiding the putty; it's in the cascade of benefits that flow from that single, elegant scan.

It's a Time Machine: The minutes of mouth-propped-open discomfort have evaporated into seconds of effortless scanning. The instant the scan is done, the model is ready. There's no waiting for plaster to set, no shipping fragile models to a lab. This speed isn't just about convenience; it's about respect for your time. It transforms a dental visit from a day-long disruption into an efficient, streamlined experience.

It's a Comfort Revolution: This is, without a doubt, the part patients celebrate the most. No goo, no taste, no pressure. For anyone with dental anxiety or a sensitive gag reflex, the IOS is more than a tool; it's a key that unlocks access to care they may have been avoiding for years. It turns a moment of dread into one of genuine curiosity.

It's Flawlessly Fluent: Traditional plaster models were like a message passed through a game of telephone—prone to tiny errors at every step. Alginate could shrink, plaster could bubble, and a model could chip in transit. A digital scan, however, is a direct, uncorrupted translation of you. It's a perfect, pristine record, ensuring that whatever is created—from a single crown to a full set of aligners—is crafted with microscopic precision for a flawless fit. This digital integrity isn't just about better outcomes; it's about getting it right the very first time.

The Scanner That Sees the Invisible

But the story doesn't end with a 3D model. The most advanced intraoral scanners have become powerful diagnostic partners, revealing secrets that were once hidden from view.

Think of it as having dental superpowers. Some scanners use special fluorescent light to illuminate early-stage cavities long before they'd show up on an X-ray or be visible to the naked eye. This is a seismic shift from reactive to proactive care, allowing dentists to stop decay in its tracks with minimally invasive treatments.

Even more profoundly, the IOS is a historian of your health. By overlaying scans from different appointments, it creates a time-lapse movie of your mouth. It can reveal the subtle erosion from nighttime grinding, track a receding gum line with millimeter precision, or spot the slightest shift in tooth alignment. These are changes that are often imperceptible during a routine exam but become glaringly obvious on screen.

This isn't just data; it's empowerment. When you can see the tiny changes happening in your own mouth, the conversation with your dentist changes. You're no longer a passive patient; you're an active, informed collaborator in your own health journey.

The First Word in a Digital Conversation

Everything that follows in modern, digital dentistry begins here. This initial, impeccable scan is the foundation upon which everything else is built. It's the source code for virtual treatment simulations, where you can see your future smile before treatment even starts. It's the digital command sent to a 3D printer that fabricates your perfectly customized aligners. It's the common language that allows your dentist, the lab technician, and other specialists to collaborate seamlessly.

The intraoral scanner has done more than just replace an unpleasant procedure. It has fundamentally changed the feeling of dentistry. It has made it faster, more comfortable, and infinitely more precise. It has turned the dental chair into a place of discovery and co-creation, where the first step to a healthier, more confident smile is no longer a mouthful of goop, but a brilliant flash of light.

The Soul of the Smile: An Artist's Journey in a Digital World

Every smile holds a unique story, a masterpiece waiting to be revealed. For generations, the tools to unlock that masterpiece were approximations—plaster casts that felt like relics and a process of educated guesswork. But today, orthodontics has found its soul in the digital realm. We've traded messy impressions for beams of light and trial-and-error for a breathtakingly precise art form. This is the story of how your perfect smile is no longer just hoped for, but meticulously designed, sculpted, and brought to life.

From a Whisper of Light to a Digital Soul

The journey begins not with a mouthful of cold, goopy paste, but with the gentle sweep of a magic wand. An intraoral scanner, glowing with soft light, dances across your teeth, capturing every curve and contour in seconds. It's a weightless, comfortable experience, but what's happening on the screen is profound. A shimmering, three-dimensional twin of your smile materializes from a cloud of data points, a perfect digital ghost of your physical self. This isn't just a model; it's the raw marble, the untouched clay from which your future smile will be sculpted. This digital soul, in formats like STL or PLY, is the first step into the artist's studio.

The Digital Studio: Where Science Becomes Art

Welcome to the orthodontist's creative sanctuary. The specialized CAD software we use is less like a computer program and more like a high-tech artist's loft, where intuition and decades of knowledge meet the limitless power of the digital canvas. Here, your digital smile can be turned, examined, and understood with a depth that plaster models could only dream of.

This is where we become architects of the bite, analyzing the intricate dance between your upper and lower teeth to ensure they meet in perfect harmony. We can peer beneath the surface, integrating scans of the roots and bone to understand the very foundation of your smile. It's a holistic view that respects the biology of your body, ensuring every planned movement is not just beautiful, but safe and lasting. In this studio, we don't just see teeth; we see the intricate, living system that is your smile.

The Liberation: Setting Each Tooth Free

Before a sculptor can reposition the arm of a statue, it must be seen as separate from the stone. In the same way, the first crucial act in our digital studio is "segmentation"—the moment of liberation. With surgical precision, the software, guided by the clinician's expert eye, digitally separates each tooth from its neighbors.

In an instant, each tooth becomes its own entity, a free spirit unshackled from the digital arch. This act of digital freedom is the key that unlocks true personalization. Now, we can choreograph the movement of a single incisor or rotate an individual molar without disturbing the rest of the symphony. This is where mass treatment ends and your unique journey begins.

The Blueprint of a Masterpiece: The Virtual Setup

This is the heart of the entire process—the moment of pure creation. The "virtual setup" is where the orthodontist, as both artist and engineer, composes your ideal smile. Guided by the principles of facial aesthetics and biomechanics, we embark on a delicate digital ballet. We gently nudge teeth into perfect alignment, close gaps, and center the smile to create a look that is uniquely, authentically you.

It's an iterative dance of making a change, viewing it from every conceivable angle, and refining it until the result is flawless. This isn't just about straight teeth; it's about crafting the graceful curve of the smile, the confident flow from one tooth to the next, and the functional harmony that will serve you for a lifetime. This final, perfected 3D model is the definitive blueprint, the North Star that will guide every step of the treatment to come.

The Journey Home: Charting the Course for Aligners

For those on the path of clear aligners, the blueprint is just the beginning. The software now becomes a brilliant time traveler, working backward from the final masterpiece. It deconstructs the entire transformation into a series of tiny, incremental steps—a finely choreographed sequence of movements.

Each step is a whisper, a gentle nudge from a custom-made aligner. If a tooth needs to travel 3mm, its journey is broken into 30 micro-movements, each one precisely programmed. The software also dictates where tiny, tooth-colored "attachments" will act as anchors, giving the aligners the leverage to perform their magic. It's a roadmap to your new smile, where every stage is planned with such incredible detail that the outcome is not just a hope, but a predictable reality.

The Power of Precision: Elevating Braces to an Art Form

Even for the timeless strength of traditional braces, this digital blueprint is revolutionary. The ideal placement of each bracket is the secret to an efficient and precise outcome. In the virtual world, we can place each bracket onto your perfected smile blueprint with micron-level accuracy.

This digital precision is then transferred to the real world through "indirect bonding trays"—custom guides that allow us to place the physical brackets on your teeth in the exact same ideal position. It's like using a perfect stencil to paint a masterpiece, ensuring the foundation of your treatment is flawless from the very first day. This method transforms the application of braces from a manual skill into a digitally-guided science, saving you time and ensuring a more predictable path to perfection.

A Glimpse of the Horizon: The Future is Personal

The artist's studio is about to get a holographic upgrade. The evolution of this technology is expanding into realms we once only dreamed of. Artificial intelligence is emerging not as a replacement, but as a wise digital consultant, offering insights from thousands of successful masterpieces to help inform the initial design.

Soon, we won't just look at a 3D model on a screen. Imagine your orthodontist walking through your treatment plan in an immersive virtual reality environment to perfect every detail. Or picture yourself, using augmented reality, to "try on" your future smile, seeing it superimposed on your own face in the mirror before the first aligner is ever worn.

This digital revolution has transformed orthodontics. It has elevated the practice from a craft into a sublime fusion of art and science, allowing us to deliver a level of personalized, predictable, and beautiful care that was once impossible. It ensures that the story your smile tells is the exact masterpiece you were always meant to share.

The Orthodontist's New Magic Wand: Forging Smiles in-House with 3D Printing

Forget what you thought you knew about getting braces or retainers. The days of goopy impressions, long waits, and the mysterious, far-off dental lab are fading into memory. There's a revolution happening, and it's not happening in a massive factory—it's humming quietly in your local orthodontist's office. It's the shift from being a customer of a production line to becoming the architect of the smile itself. Welcome to the age of in-office 3D printing, where orthodontists are trading in their prescription pads for design files and becoming creators.

This isn't just about a new gadget in the corner; it's a fundamental change in the entire philosophy of care. It's the difference between ordering a suit and having a master tailor right in the room with you, stitching a perfectly bespoke garment on the spot.

The Two Spells of Creation: A Tale of Light and Liquid

At the heart of this new workshop are two fascinating technologies that sound like something out of a sci-fi novel: Stereolithography (SLA) and Digital Light Processing (DLP). Both are a kind of modern alchemy, transforming a liquid photopolymer resin into a solid, precise dental device. They literally build smiles out of light and liquid.

Imagine an artist. SLA is like a master painter with a single, incredibly fine brush—a laser. This laser meticulously traces every detail of a single layer onto the surface of the resin, hardening it with pinpoint accuracy. It then moves on, layer by whisper-thin layer, building the object with breathtaking precision. This method is the champion of detail, creating appliances with a glassy-smooth finish, perfect for the most intricate and demanding jobs where every single micron is a universe of its own.

Now, picture a different kind of artist. DLP is like a master of stencils and light. Instead of a single point of light, it uses a digital projector to flash the image of an entire layer all at once, like a camera flash freezing a moment in time. Flash. An entire slice of the retainer is cured. Flash. The next layer is born. This makes DLP the speed demon of the duo. It's the go-to for a busy practice that needs to produce multiple appliances, turning the office into a high-throughput studio for smile creation. While SLA once held the crown for detail, DLP technology is advancing so rapidly that for many orthodontic needs, the difference is virtually invisible—but the speed is undeniable.

The In-House Creation Station: What's on the Menu?

So, what exactly are these newly empowered orthodontists creating? The applications are as broad as the orthodontist's imagination.

Same-Day Retainers: The End of the Anxious Wait

This is perhaps the most immediate "wow" moment for patients. Picture it: the braces are finally off! The teeth are free! In the old world, this moment was tinged with anxiety. You'd have a new impression taken and be sent home to wait for a week, maybe two, for your retainers to arrive from a lab. In that gap, those newly freed teeth could start their subtle, rebellious drift back to their old positions. With in-house 3D printing, that gap vanishes. A quick, comfortable digital scan of your new smile is sent directly to the printer. Before you've even finished scrolling through your social media feed, a perfectly clear, custom-fit retainer is printed, cured, and ready to take home. You walk out of the office on the same day with the insurance policy for your new smile already in hand.

The In-House Aligner Revolution

Clear aligners have changed the face of orthodontics, but they often come with a brand name and a hefty price tag. In-house 3D printing hands the keys to the kingdom back to the orthodontist. They can now design and print an entire series of custom aligners right in the office. This "vertical integration" not only makes treatment more affordable but allows for incredible agility. Lost an aligner?

No problem. A new one can be printed that afternoon, keeping your treatment perfectly on track. It allows the orthodontist to be the director, producer, and editor of your smile journey, from the first frame to the last.

Indirect Bonding Trays: Placing Brackets with Digital Perfection

This is where the technology becomes truly transformative for the clinician. Placing brackets on teeth is a delicate art, and perfect placement is the key to efficient and predictable treatment. 3D printing allows for the creation of "indirect bonding trays." First, the orthodontist uses sophisticated software to place the brackets on a virtual 3D model of your teeth in their absolute, geometrically perfect positions. Then, they 3D print a flexible, custom tray that fits over your teeth, holding each of those brackets in its pre-planned, perfect spot. In the clinic, the orthodontist simply fills the tray with adhesive, places it in your mouth, and voilà—every bracket is transferred to its ideal location at once. It's a level of precision that is nearly impossible to achieve by hand, leading to better results and often shorter treatment times.

More Than a Machine: The Dawn of the Creator Practice

When you bring manufacturing in-house, you're doing more than just saving on lab fees. You're fundamentally changing the rhythm and potential of your practice.

Goodbye, Waiting Games: Turnaround times that were once measured in weeks are now measured in hours. This immediacy means treatment never stalls, and patients are happier.

Embracing Agility: The orthodontist can now pivot on a dime. If a treatment plan needs a slight tweak, a new model or appliance can be fabricated instantly. It's like having a creative sandbox where solutions can be tested and implemented without delay.

A Symphony of Customization: Every appliance is born from a patient's unique digital blueprint, leading to a level of fit and comfort that was once a luxury.

The Patient Experience, Reimagined: The journey becomes faster, more comfortable (no more gag-inducing impressions!), and more engaging. Patients feel like they are part of a cutting-edge process, which builds trust and excitement.

Of course, stepping into this new role requires an investment—not just in equipment, but in learning. There's a new language of design software to speak, and a new craft of printer operation to master. But for practices willing to embrace the learning curve, the rewards are immense.

The future isn't coming; it's already here, glowing in vats of resin and humming in practices around the world. The shift from gatekeeper to creator is redefining what it means to be an orthodontist, empowering them with the tools to deliver care that is more precise, agile, and wonderfully human than ever before.

The Siren Song of the Shortcut Smile: A Reality Check on DIY Orthodontics

In the glow of your screen, it seems so simple, so seductive. A world of perfect smiles, seemingly unlocked with a YouTube tutorial and a 3D printer humming in the corner of your room. The internet whispers a tempting promise: "Why pay a fortune? Why wait for appointments? Take control. Do it yourself." It's the ultimate life hack, applied to the very landscape of your face. But before you download that file, before you mix that resin, we need to talk. Not as a textbook lecturing you, but as someone who understands the pull of a shortcut and has seen the wreckage at the end of that perilous path.

This isn't about shaming your ingenuity or your desire for a more confident smile. It's about pulling back the curtain on a dangerous illusion. Because straightening your teeth isn't like building a spice rack or knitting a scarf. You're not working with wood or yarn; you're attempting to command the living, breathing architecture of your own body. This isn't a DIY project; it's amateur surgery on the dining room table, and the consequences can be devastatingly permanent.

Your Smile is a Living System, Not a Set of Dominoes

To understand the gamble you're taking, you have to see your teeth not as simple pegs to be pushed into line, but as living entities deeply rooted in a dynamic ecosystem. An orthodontic aligner isn't a passive plastic tray; it's a prescription-strength tool designed to command a slow, deliberate biological symphony.

Picture each tooth anchored in your jaw by a living tether—the periodontal ligament. This web of fibers is a marvel of natural engineering, a sensitive network that responds to every force. When a professionally guided force is applied, it's like a gentle, persuasive conversation with your body. On one side of the root, specialized cells are signaled to clear away a sliver of bone, making space. On the other side, different cells get the message to build new bone, securing the tooth in its new home. It's a delicate, microscopic process of demolition and construction, happening in perfect harmony.

A DIY device, however, is a sledgehammer in this delicate construction zone. It applies brute, uninformed force. It doesn't whisper; it shouts. And your body, under that kind of duress, doesn't remodel. It panics.

The Ghost in the Machine: The Horrors You Can't See Coming

The real tragedy of DIY orthodontics is that the worst damage happens out of sight, deep beneath the gum line, only revealing itself when it's far too late.

Imagine the roots of your teeth, the very foundation of your smile, literally dissolving under the pressure. This is severe root resorption, and it's a silent, insidious thief. The uncontrolled forces from a poorly made aligner can cause your body to eat away at its own tooth structure. The roots shorten, becoming brittle, fragile stumps. Your teeth might look straighter for a fleeting moment, but they are standing on a crumbling foundation, primed for a future of loosening, fracture, and ultimately, loss. Once that root is gone, it's gone forever. You can't 3D print a new one.

Then there's the slow, painful creep of gum recession. As your gums pull away from the tooth in retreat from the traumatic forces, they expose the sensitive, vulnerable roots. This isn't just a cosmetic issue; it's an open invitation for a lifetime of sharp, shocking pain, relentless decay, and advanced gum disease. Restoring lost gum tissue is a painful, expensive, and often uncertain surgical ordeal.

And let's not forget your jaw joint, the TMJ. It's the complex hinge that lets you talk, eat, and laugh. Proper orthodontics creates a bite where everything works in harmony. DIY orthodontics can slam your teeth together into a dysfunctional, clashing mess, putting immense strain on this delicate joint. The result? Chronic headaches, a jaw that clicks and pops, agonizing pain, and even the terrifying sensation of your jaw locking shut. Your quest for a prettier smile could end with you unable to enjoy a simple meal.

The Professional's Touch: More Than Just a Straightener of Teeth

An orthodontist is not just a provider of braces. They are a biomechanical architect, a medical diagnostician, and a guardian of your oral health. Their journey begins not with an impression tray, but with a deep, investigative look into your unique anatomy. X-rays reveal the unseen story—the length and health of your roots, the density of your bone, the presence of impacted teeth that could turn your DIY project into a disaster.

They don't just see crooked teeth; they see the intricate relationship between your teeth, your jaw, and your entire facial structure. Their treatment plan is a personalized blueprint, meticulously designed to respect the limits of your biology. They use FDA-approved, biocompatible materials that won't poison you or shatter in your mouth. Every adjustment is a deliberate, monitored step in a carefully choreographed dance. They are your safety net, constantly watching for the slightest sign of trouble and intervening before it becomes a catastrophe.

In a world obsessed with instant gratification and technological empowerment, it is a radical act of self-care to recognize the limits of our own expertise. 3D printing is a revolutionary tool, but in the realm of medicine, its power belongs in the hands of a trained, licensed, and accountable professional.

So, please, step away from the allure of the quick fix. Your smile is not a trend to be hacked or a project to be trialed. It's a precious, living part of you, deserving of respect and expert care. An investment in professional orthodontics isn't just an investment in straight teeth; it's an investment in a future of healthy gums, strong bones, and a confident, pain-free smile that will truly last a lifetime. Don't let your story become a cautionary tale whispered in online forums. Choose the path of wisdom. Your future self will thank you.

The Science and Biomechanics of Clear Aligner Therapy

The Secret Life of a Smile: The Silent Dance of Clear Aligners

Your future smile has a secret. It's not forged in steel or announced with a glint of metal. It begins with a whisper. A nearly invisible, perfectly planned whisper that coaxes your teeth into a new reality. This is the world of clear aligners, and their magic isn't magic at all—it's a silent, intimate dance between your body and one of the most intelligent materials ever created for a smile.

Forget the word "plastic." Think of your aligner as a memory keeper. It's crafted from a special kind of thermoplastic, a material with a past and a future. In the lab, under precise heat, it becomes impressionable, like warm wax. It's then molded into a vision—not of your teeth as they are, but as they will be in two weeks. As it cools, this vision solidifies, locking in the memory of your next step towards a perfect smile. When you first snap a new aligner into place, it feels snug for a reason: you are introducing your teeth to their own future.

The Persistent Push: A Muscle Made of Memory

The true genius of an aligner lives in its relentless desire to return to that original, perfect shape. This is its elasticity. Imagine pressing your hand into a memory foam pillow. The moment you lift it, the foam begins to rise, tirelessly seeking its original form. Your aligner does the same thing.

From the moment it envelops your teeth, it's fighting to spring back to the shape it was born with. This isn't a harsh shove or a forceful yank. It's a continuous, gentle pressure—a constant, unwavering suggestion. This light, persistent force is the biological secret to unlocking tooth movement. It's a quiet conversation, a constant nudge telling the cells in your jawbone, "It's time to remodel, time to make way for something new." Without this energetic memory, the aligner would just be a passive mouthguard, and your smile's journey would never begin.

The Battle Against Forgetting: An Aligner's Race Against Time

But even the most dedicated memory can fade. The same way a new pair of leather shoes eventually softens and loses its initial, rigid shape, an aligner faces a formidable challenge: stress relaxation. Think of it as material fatigue. As the aligner tirelessly applies its gentle force, it's also adapting to the reality of your teeth. It can get a little too comfortable in its stretched position, and the force it delivers can begin to wane.

This is why an ideal aligner is a paradox: it must be flexible enough to move your teeth, yet stubborn enough to resist "forgetting" its mission. Manufacturers wage a constant war against this tendency, designing materials that can hold their tension and keep whispering their instructions for the full one- or two-week journey. Your orthodontist isn't just giving you a new aligner every couple of weeks; they are giving you a fresh soldier with a perfect memory, ready to pick up the dance where the last one left off.

The Difference Between a Hug and a Poke

The way an aligner delivers its message is profoundly different from the old-school approach. Traditional braces are like a series of specific pressure points, poking and pulling on a tooth with a wire. An aligner, however, delivers a full-body hug.

By completely enveloping the visible part of the tooth, it applies its force across a vast surface area. This embrace has a powerful biomechanical advantage. Consider moving a tooth deeper into the bone—a movement orthodontists call intrusion. Trying to do this with braces can be like trying to push a bowling pin straight down by poking it in the side; it's more likely to tip. But the aligner's hug allows it to apply a gentle, downward pressure along the tooth's entire axis. It's the difference between a nudge and a direct, confident guide, allowing for movements that were once incredibly complex to become predictable and efficient.

The Tiny Battlefield of Your Mouth

We can design the perfect material in a sterile lab, but its true test comes when it enters the chaotic world of your mouth. The oral cavity is a warm, wet, and wild environment, constantly changing with every sip of coffee, every bite of a lemon, and every passing microbe.

Studies that look at aligners after their two-week tour of duty reveal a hidden story of survival. Under a microscope, the once-pristine surface shows battle scars—microscopic roughness and signs of wear from this constant exposure. This isn't just cosmetic. This subtle degradation can impact how the aligner performs, potentially dampening the very forces it was designed to deliver. It's a stark reminder that these are high-performance instruments on a short, intense mission.

Understanding this dance—the material's memory, its inevitable fatigue, its full-embrace force, and its battle for survival in your mouth—is the first step to mastering the art of clear aligner therapy. It allows your orthodontist to be more than a doctor; it makes them a choreographer, planning each two-week step with breathtaking precision.

So the next time you hold a clear aligner, know that you're not just holding a piece of plastic. You're holding a memory. A silent, invisible mover, custom-built to have a two-week conversation with your body, patiently and persistently guiding you toward the smile you've always imagined.

The Secret Handholds of a Perfect Smile

We all understand the dream: a smile that feels like coming home, effortless and bright. For a long time, the path to that smile was a river of steel—traditional braces, effective but obvious. Then, a new current emerged: clear aligners. These whispered promises of a gentler, invisible journey. Like a smooth, clear stone skipping across water, they seemed to nudge our teeth into place with quiet grace.

And for the simple journeys, they were perfect. A slight tilt here, a small shift there. The aligner, a sleek, transparent guide, would press against the polished enamel of a tooth, and the tooth would listen. It was a simple conversation.

But our bodies are rarely simple. They are intricate landscapes of stunning complexity. What happens when a tooth is not just leaning, but has turned its back on the world? What if it's hiding shyly in the gums, or needs to be guided deeper to find its foundation? What if the very root, the anchor beneath the surface, needs to pivot?

This is where the simple, skipping stone sinks. Imagine trying to scale a sheer cliff face of polished marble. It might be beautiful, but your hands find no purchase. There's no grip, no leverage, no way to do anything but slide. The smooth, elegant surface of a tooth presents the very same challenge to a simple aligner. For the complex, acrobatic movements required for a truly masterful smile, the aligner needs something to hold onto.

This is where the magic happens. This is where your orthodontist becomes a master route-setter, and your teeth become the face of a mountain about to be climbed.

The Climber's Holds: What Attachments Truly Are

Enter the unsung heroes of your aligner journey: attachments. Forget clinical descriptions. Think of them as tiny, bespoke sculptures—or better yet, as custom-designed climbing holds bonded directly to your teeth. They are crafted from a composite resin that is color-matched to your enamel, like a chameleon, making them remarkably discreet.

The process of placing them is less a procedure and more an act of artistry. Your orthodontist, the route-setter, uses a precise template to place these tiny resin forms onto specific teeth. A beam of light hardens them in an instant, and suddenly, the smooth, impossible cliff face has handholds. They are painless, unassuming, and they change everything.

How Tiny Shapes Become Giants of Force

So how do these little bumps, these subtle new shapes, accomplish so much? They transform the conversation between your aligner and your tooth.

Before, the aligner could only push. It was a monologue. Now, with an attachment, the aligner has a dance partner.

Your aligner is created with a perfect little pocket, a custom-made indentation that 'clicks' over the attachment. It's a lock-and-key system. This connection is the secret. It's the grip that allows the aligner to stop just pushing and start orchestrating a delicate dance of pressure and release. It can now create leverage.

Think of the climber on that cliff. With a hold, they can not only push, but pull, twist, and anchor themselves to perform incredible feats. In the same way, the aligner uses the attachment to:

Master Rotation: A stubborn, rounded tooth is like a spinning ball. It's nearly impossible to grip. But with a small, rectangular attachment, the aligner now has two distinct surfaces to push and pull against. It creates a "turning force," a gentle, relentless torque that can spin a rotated tooth perfectly into line, like a dancer completing a pirouette.

Conquer Extrusion: Trying to pull a tooth further out of the gumline with a smooth aligner is like trying to lift a wet bar of soap. It will just slip away. But an attachment acts as a tiny ledge or "undercut." The aligner can now "hook" onto this surface, applying a steady, upward pull that coaxes the tooth into its rightful place.

Perfect Torque (The Root of the Matter): This is the most profound movement of all—guiding the root of the tooth. It's like moving the foundation of a house. For this, an attachment acts as a sophisticated lever. The aligner will press on the attachment near the gumline while simultaneously pressing on the upper part of the tooth. This creates a twisting, "torquing" force that pivots the root through the bone, a movement that is absolutely critical for a stable, healthy bite and a visually perfect result. It's the difference between a temporary fix and a lifelong foundation.

The Art and Soul of the Plan

None of this is guesswork. The shape, size, and placement of every single attachment is part of a grand, digital blueprint. Using breathtakingly powerful software, your orthodontist can simulate the entire journey. They can become a digital rock-climbing choreographer, testing every hold, every pressure point, and every potential path in a virtual world before the first aligner is ever printed. This fusion of biomechanical science and clinical artistry ensures that your journey is not just hopeful, but predictable.

When you first get your attachments, your tongue will be a curious explorer, mapping these new little bumps. But within a day or two, they become a seamless part of you. And when your journey is complete, when you have reached the summit, they are polished away without a trace, as if they were never there.

The only evidence of their existence is the breathtaking view: your new smile.

Attachments are the silent partners to the clear aligner. They are the reason this gentle technology can perform acts of incredible strength. They are the small, brilliant innovation that turns a simple nudge into a sophisticated dance, proving that sometimes, to achieve the most beautiful and complex goals, all you need is the right place to grip.

The Secret Choreography of Your Smile

We all know the feeling. A glance in the mirror, a photo, a moment of self-consciousness about our smile. For years, the path to changing that smile was a very visible one, paved with metal brackets and wires. But today, clear aligners have changed the game, offering a journey that's discreet, flexible, and almost invisible.

But the magic isn't in the clear plastic itself. The aligner is just the tool. The real artistry, the genius behind every breathtaking smile transformation, is the secret story written before your first aligner is ever worn. It's a detailed choreography, a meticulously planned dance for your teeth, known in the orthodontic world as the digital treatment plan.

The Score for the Symphony: Your Digital Plan

Imagine a world-class choreographer preparing for a new ballet. They wouldn't just send dancers onto the stage and hope for the best. They would write a score—a detailed, step-by-step map of every movement, every leap, every turn, from the opening curtain to the final bow.

Your digital treatment plan is that score. It translates the grand finale—your perfect smile—into a series of tiny, graceful steps. Each step corresponds to a single clear aligner. You wear one, and your teeth perform the first move. You switch to the next, and they execute the second. This continues, aligner by aligner, as your smile gradually performs its beautifully choreographed routine.

The quality of this choreography is everything. A flawed score can lead to a clumsy performance, with dancers bumping into each other or missing their marks. A brilliant one ensures every movement is efficient, safe, and leads to a stunning, harmonious result. The success of your entire journey hinges on the artistry and foresight embedded in this initial plan.

The Group Number: Staging the Big Picture

To appreciate the genius of this plan, we have to look at it through two lenses. The first is the "group number"—the grand, sweeping movements that involve your entire dental arch. This is the choreographer's vision for the whole troupe of dancers on stage.

This involves asking critical questions about the performance as a whole. For instance, does the entire stage (your arch) need to be widened first, giving the dancers more room before they begin their individual, intricate steps? Or can they expand their formation while simultaneously performing? The sequence is crucial. Creating space first can unlock movements that would otherwise be impossible.

This is also where the choreographer decides on the "anchors" of the performance. In any complex dance, some dancers must remain perfectly still, providing a stable core that others can move against. In your mouth, some teeth must be designated as anchors to allow others to move predictably. Without this stability, the whole performance could become chaotic.

Finally, the group number addresses a fundamental question: how do we create space on a crowded stage? If your teeth are crowded, the plan must make room. This can be achieved through several elegant techniques:

A Little Breathing Room: Gently polishing away a whisper-thin layer of enamel between teeth, a technique called Interproximal Reduction (IPR), can create just enough space for dancers to move without bumping elbows.

A Step Forward or Back: The entire line of front teeth can be guided slightly forward or backward to create a new, more spacious arrangement.

Moving the Back Row: The rearmost teeth can be gently guided further back, opening up the stage in front of them.

Casting Call: In very crowded situations, removing a tooth might be like recasting a role to give the stars of the show the space they need to truly shine.

These big-picture decisions create the foundation and flow for the entire masterpiece.

The Soloists: Perfecting Each Tooth's Performance

While the group number sets the stage, the magic is also in the "solo performances"—the incredibly detailed choreography for each individual tooth. This is where the biomechanical artistry truly comes alive.

Imagine two dancers standing shoulder-to-shoulder. You can't ask one to perform a wild spin without first creating a pocket of space. The plan for each tooth must be perfectly compatible with its neighbors, preventing any "collisions" or "binding." The choreography might dictate that one tooth takes a small step aside before its partner begins a complex rotation.

This micro-level planning prioritizes movements to make others possible. Difficult steps like a "lift" (pulling a tooth out, or extrusion) or a deep "plié" (pushing a tooth into the bone, or intrusion) require immense precision. The digital plan doesn't just show the final position; it dictates the exact path and force needed for every single step of the journey, ensuring the performance is both beautiful and safe.

The Choreographer's Eye: The Orthodontist's New Superpower

In the age of digital orthodontics, the orthodontist's role has evolved from a skilled craftsman bending wires to a master choreographer with a new superpower: digital biomechanical literacy.

This isn't about computer coding. It's about having the soul of an artist and the mind of an engineer. Sophisticated software can generate a dance routine, but it can't feel the music. A computer can propose a sequence of movements, but it doesn't have the real-world experience to know if a move is too ambitious or if it ignores the subtle physics of the human body.

An orthodontist with this literacy can look at a digital plan and see the story behind the data. They can spot where a proposed movement, while looking perfect on screen, might be clunky or unpredictable in reality. They understand that for every action, there is an equal and opposite reaction in your mouth, and they ensure this delicate balance is respected. They are the human soul that transforms a computer's suggestion into a clinical masterpiece.

The Director's Notes: The Art of the Perfect Adjustment

A great choreographer never just accepts the first draft. They refine it, tweak it, and elevate it. This is where the orthodontist's expertise becomes your treatment's greatest asset. They modify the initial plan with a series of brilliant adjustments:

Adding Handholds (Attachments): An aligner is smooth, and so is a tooth. Trying to get a good grip for a complex move, like rotating a round tooth, can be like trying to turn a wet doorknob. Attachments—tiny, tooth-colored bumps—are the solution. They act like a partner's strategically placed hand, giving the aligner a firm "grip" to execute a difficult lift or spin with grace and precision.

Re-Choreographing the Sequence: Instead of having every dancer move at once, which can lead to chaos, the orthodontist might segment the performance. They might have the back row of teeth move first, establishing a strong foundation, and then cue the front teeth to begin their more delicate and visible routine. This improves control and ensures the performance never goes off track.

Planning for the Encore (Overcorrection): This is a stroke of genius born from experience. A great dancer often pushes a final pose just a little further, knowing it will settle into a position of perfect, relaxed grace. Similarly, an orthodontist might plan for a tooth to move slightly beyond its final destination. This builds in a buffer, accounting for the natural tendency of teeth to settle back a tiny bit. This "overcorrection" ensures that when your treatment is over, your teeth settle into their truly flawless positions, rather than falling just short.

The Standing Ovation

Your clear aligner journey is so much more than a series of plastic trays. It is a work of performance art, a symphony of movement composed and conducted just for you. It is a partnership between the elegant science of biomechanics and the intuitive artistry of an experienced orthodontist.

This is the new world of orthodontics. It's about mastering technology, but more importantly, it's about understanding how to use it to choreograph a smile that is not only beautiful and healthy but is ready for its standing ovation.

The Aligner & The Dance: A Guide to Your Smile's New Moves

Think of starting clear aligner therapy not as a medical procedure, but as learning a new dance. You have a partner—the aligner—and a goal: a beautifully choreographed smile. Your orthodontist is the expert choreographer, designing every step. And you? You are the star dancer.

This dance is sleek, modern, and almost invisible to the audience. That's its magic. But like any intricate performance, some moves are simple and flowing, while others are complex lifts and spins that require perfect technique, extra support, and unwavering dedication.

The music starts with a digital "map" of the entire dance, often called a ClinCheck. It's a stunning preview of the final bow. But here's the secret every great dancer knows: the rehearsal rarely looks exactly like the blueprint. In the real world, the overall accuracy of the dance—the difference between the plan and the final result—hovers around 50-67%. This isn't a sign of failure; it's the nature of the dance. It means the partnership between you, your orthodontist, and your aligners is a dynamic, living process.

The Simple, Flowing Steps (The Highly Predictable Moves)

These are the foundational moves your aligner partner leads with confidence and grace.

The Gentle Lean (Tilting): Imagine gently swaying a tooth toward your lip or back toward your tongue. This is your aligner's favorite move. The plastic fits snugly over the crown, giving it a broad surface to press against. It's a straightforward, elegant nudge that aligners perform with beautiful precision.

The Subtle Dip (Minor Intrusion): For your front teeth, a slight push upward into the gumline is a relatively simple maneuver. The aligner has a good grip and can effectively guide your incisors into a more harmonious position.

The Forward-and-Back Rock (Tipping Along the Arch): Tilting a tooth forward or backward in line with your smile is another move that's well within your aligner's comfort zone. Tipping is always easier than moving the entire tooth, and aligners handle this with reliable poise.

The Advanced Choreography (The Challenging Moves)

This is where your choreographer's expertise truly shines. These ambitious moves are possible, but they require special preparation, extra tools, and a flawless performance from you.

The Dramatic Lift (Extrusion): Coaxing a tooth out of the bone is the most challenging move in the entire performance. It's like a dramatic lift in a ballet. The aligner, being smooth plastic, can struggle to get a firm enough grip to pull the tooth downward. It often wants to slip. Without help, the accuracy can be as low as 30%. To nail this lift, your choreographer will bond special "grips" (attachments) to the tooth and may even call in for extra support from tiny "wires" (elastics) to ensure the tooth moves with power and grace.

The Pirouette (Rotating Round Teeth): Trying to spin a round tooth, like a canine or premolar, is like trying to turn a doorknob with a flat hand. There's not enough to grab onto! The aligner can easily slip. For these tricky rotations, especially anything more than a slight turn, success depends entirely on "costuming." Your orthodontist will add strategically shaped attachments that give the aligner the leverage it needs to complete the spin.

Shifting Your Center of Gravity (Root Movement & Torque): Tipping a tooth's crown is one thing; moving the entire root through the bone is another challenge altogether. This is the difference between leaning and taking a full, controlled step. It requires a sophisticated application of force that tests the limits of what a plastic aligner can do on its own. While the crown might move, getting the root to follow perfectly is where we often see a gap between the plan and the reality.

The Supporting Cast: What Makes the Dance a Success

No performance is a solo act. The success of your smile's transformation relies on a dedicated team and the right tools.

Your Choreographer (The Orthodontist): An experienced orthodontist doesn't just press "play" on the digital plan. They read it like a composer reads a score, anticipating the difficult passages. They know precisely when to add an attachment, call for elastics, or even plan for more movement than needed (a technique called "overcorrection") to ensure the final result is perfect.

The "Costume" and "Props" (Attachments & Auxiliaries): Those little bumps bonded to your teeth (attachments) are not flaws; they are the custom-fit grips on your dance costume, essential for the difficult lifts and spins. Elastics and other aids are the props that can turn a challenging move into a stunning success.

Your Dedication (Patient Compliance): Here is the most critical part: you are the dancer. The aligner is your partner, but it can't dance alone. If the choreographer asks for 22 hours of rehearsal a day, that's what it takes. Skipping wear time is like missing practice before opening night—the entire performance can falter. Your commitment is the single most important factor in bringing the choreography to life.

The Final Bow

Choosing clear aligners is choosing a specific, beautiful style of dance. It's a partnership that can create breathtaking results. By understanding where your partner is strong and where it needs support, you can set realistic expectations. You'll know that the journey may require a few extra rehearsals (refinements) and some special tools along the way.

With a skilled choreographer guiding you and your own dedication to the performance, you are destined for a spectacular final bow: a healthy, confident smile that was worth every step of the dance.

Accelerating Orthodontic Treatment: A Critical Review of Current Evidence

The Secret Conversation: How Your Body Can Fast-Track Your Smile

Imagine your body has a secret language. It's a language of action, a constant, quiet conversation of healing and rebuilding that happens without you even thinking about it. When you scrape your knee, a silent alarm sounds, and a flood of microscopic medics rushes to the scene. But what if we could learn to speak that language? What if we could ask your body to focus its incredible healing power on one specific goal?

This is the beautiful idea behind a remarkable biological process, and it's changing the face of orthodontics. It's called the Regional Acceleratory Phenomenon (RAP), but it's easier to think of it as a secret superpower locked inside your bones, just waiting for the right password.

Waking the Giant: The Story of RAP

Decades ago, a visionary surgeon named Harold Frost was listening closely to the body's secrets. He was a master of understanding bone, and he noticed something extraordinary. When a bone was nudged—through an injury, a fracture, or even a deliberate surgical tap—it didn't just patch itself up. It woke up.

In the precise area of that nudge, the body would unleash a tidal wave of focused energy. It was like a sleeping giant stirred to life, suddenly alive with activity. Frost realized this wasn't just simple repair; it was an accelerated, supercharged healing event. This is RAP: a temporary, hyper-local biological festival thrown by your body to rebuild and fortify an area with breathtaking speed.

The Dream Team of Renovation

So, what happens when this healing festival kicks off? Your body calls in its elite renovation crew. This team has two star players:

The Demolition Experts (Osteoclasts): Think of these cells as the masters of creative destruction. Their job is to clear out the old, tired, and compromised bone tissue. During RAP, they don't just show up; they swarm the site, working with incredible efficiency to make way for the new.

The Master Builders (Osteoblasts): Following right behind the demolition team are the artisans. These are the cells that spin the fresh, strong web of new bone. They are the builders who lay the foundation and construct the new reality.

Normally, this demolition and construction process is a slow, steady dance. But when RAP is activated, the music speeds up. The dance becomes a whirlwind of activity. The crew works overtime, remodeling the bone at a pace that is simply not possible under normal circumstances.

The Golden Window: Softening the Landscape

Here is where the real magic happens, especially for moving teeth. As this supercharged renovation crew gets to work, something fascinating occurs. For a short period, the demolition team works slightly faster than the building team. This creates a temporary state where the bone in that specific area becomes softer, more porous, and less dense.

This isn't a weakness. It's a window of opportunity.

Imagine trying to move a fence post set in hard, dry, compacted earth. It's a struggle. Now, imagine that same earth has been freshly tilled, aerated, and softened. The post can now glide through it with minimal effort.

This temporary softening of the bone—this "tilling of the soil"—is the absolute key. It creates a short-lived, pliable landscape through which your teeth can move.

The Orthodontic Partnership: Speaking the Body's Language

This is where your orthodontist becomes a partner in your body's secret conversation. Traditional orthodontics works by applying slow, steady pressure, patiently waiting for the bone to remodel. It works, but it's like convincing that hard, compacted earth to yield over years.

Accelerated orthodontics, using RAP, is like your orthodontist whispering the password to awaken the giant.

Using tiny, minimally invasive techniques—like small perforations or micro-cuts in the bone around your teeth—the orthodontist provides the gentle nudge needed to activate RAP. It's just enough of a signal to tell your body, "Hey! We need your healing superpower right here, right now!"

Your body enthusiastically responds. The healing festival begins, the renovation crew is deployed, and that golden window of soft, pliable bone opens up. Now, the gentle pressure from your braces or aligners doesn't have to fight against rigid bone. Instead, your teeth can take a smooth, express route to their new positions. The resistance is dramatically lowered, and movement happens with astonishing speed.

This supercharged state lasts for about three to four months—a precious window where the most dramatic changes happen. This is why adjustments may be more frequent; your orthodontist is making the most of this incredible biological opportunity.

It's a profound shift in thinking: from forcing change upon the body to unlocking the phenomenal power that already exists within it. By learning its language and respectfully asking for its help, modern orthodontics is proving that the journey to a brilliant smile can be a brilliant collaboration with the incredible healing machine you call your body.

The Shortcut to a Straighter Smile: Are We Hacking Our Way Through Orthodontics?

The orthodontist's chair. It's a place of hope, of progress, and for many, a place where one question echoes silently in their minds: "Are we there yet?"

The journey to a perfect smile is a marathon, not a sprint. But what if there was a way to jog a few of those miles? What if you could bio-hack your own body, sending a signal to your bones to pick up the pace? This isn't science fiction. It's the tantalizing promise behind two modern techniques: Micro-Osteoperforations (MOPs) and Piezocision.

These procedures are built on a fascinating biological secret our bodies have kept for millennia: the Regional Acceleratory Phenomenon, or RAP. Think of it as your body's elite construction crew. When a bone senses a minor, controlled injury, it doesn't just patch the hole—it overhauls the entire neighborhood. It floods the area with resources, breaking down old structures and rebuilding new ones at a supercharged rate.

MOPs and Piezocision are essentially two different ways to sound the alarm and call in that crew, hoping to create a temporary "window of opportunity" where the bone around your teeth becomes softer and more malleable, allowing them to glide into place faster. But are these techniques the superhighway to a new smile, or just a scenic route with a bit of hype?

MOPs: The Gentle Nudge

Imagine a procedure so subtle it's done right in your regular dental chair. That's the essence of Micro-Osteoperforations. MOPs is the minimalist's approach to bio-hacking.

Think of it as giving your jawbone a gentle, strategic "nudge." Using a small, vibrating handpiece, the orthodontist creates a few tiny, pin-prick-sized perforations in the bone right where you need the most movement. There are no scalpels, no stitches—just a targeted signal to wake up the bone's remodeling team.

The experience for the patient is often compared to the mild discomfort of a thorough cleaning. The goal isn't to be aggressive; it's to whisper to the bone, not shout. By creating these micro-injuries, the body's RAP response kicks in. The bone density temporarily decreases, the cellular traffic increases, and the path for your moving teeth, in theory, becomes as soft as freshly tilled soil.

Piezocision: The Ultrasonic Artist

If MOPs is a gentle nudge, Piezocision is a more deliberate, artistic stroke. It's a slightly more involved technique, but one that trades subtlety for precision.

Piezocision begins with tiny, almost invisible incisions made in the gum between the teeth. Through these small gateways, the orthodontist introduces the star of the show: a piezoelectric knife. This isn't a blade in the traditional sense. It's an ultrasonic artist. It uses high-frequency vibrations to make clean, precise cuts in the hard bone without damaging the delicate surrounding gums, nerves, or blood vessels.

These controlled bone cuts are deeper and more defined than the perforations of MOPs, designed to trigger a more robust RAP response. Afterward, a stitch or two closes the tiny incisions, and the healing—and accelerated movement—begins. It's a fusion of surgical skill and high-tech finesse, aiming for maximum effect with minimal trauma.

The Reality Check: Does the Shortcut Really Shorten the Trip?

This all sounds incredible. Faster treatment, less time in braces—who wouldn't sign up? This is where we have to move from the glossy brochure to the fine print of scientific research. When we ask the hard questions, the answers become a lot less clear.

Early excitement and promising case studies created a huge buzz around these techniques. But when scientists put them under the microscope with rigorous, large-scale reviews—the gold standard of medical evidence—the picture gets fuzzy.

Imagine trying to determine the fastest car by having them race on different tracks, with different drivers, in different weather. This is the challenge researchers face. Studies on MOPs and Piezocision are so varied in their methods that it's difficult to draw a single, solid conclusion.

What these comprehensive reviews consistently tell us is this: the evidence is shaky. While some studies do show a temporary burst of speed in tooth movement right after the procedure, it's often like a short sprint at the beginning of a marathon. The effect tends to wear off, and there's very little high-quality proof that these techniques significantly reduce the overall time you spend in treatment. A potential gain of a few weeks might be possible in some cases, but the dramatic time-slashing results patients hope for are not consistently supported by science.

The Crossroads of Choice

So, where does this leave you, the person in the chair just wanting to see your new smile in the mirror?

It leaves you at a crossroads of personal choice. MOPs and Piezocision are not snake oil; they are fascinating innovations pushing the boundaries of what's possible. But they aren't magic wands, either.

The real question becomes a very human one: Is the possibility of a slightly shorter journey worth the certainty of an extra procedure, with its associated discomfort and cost? Is a temporary speed boost at the beginning worth it if the finish line isn't much closer?

The answer lies in a candid conversation with your orthodontist—your trusted guide on this journey. They can help you weigh the slick appeal of acceleration against the scientific reality. Together, you can decide if "bio-hacking" your smile is the right path for you, or if the tried-and-true scenic route, with its predictable pace and beautiful destination, is the wisest choice after all.

The Spotlight on a Faster Smile: Is Light the Secret to Better Orthodontics?

Let's be honest. The thought of getting braces or aligners brings a mixed bag of emotions. On one hand, you're excited about the promise of a perfect, confident smile. On the other, you're bracing yourself (pun intended) for the long haul—months, even years, of appointments, adjustments, and a certain level of... well, discomfort. It's the biggest hurdle for most of us, that long and sometimes tender journey to straight teeth.

For years, the only way to speed things up involved surgical procedures, a path not many are eager to take. But what if there was a different way? What if we could nudge biology along, working with your body to make the process faster, more comfortable, and even healthier?

Enter Photobiomodulation, or PBM. It might sound like something from a sci-fi movie, but it's a remarkably gentle and deeply researched therapy that's changing the orthodontic experience. Forget invasive procedures; PBM uses the simple, healing power of light to transform your treatment from a marathon into a more manageable sprint.

Giving Your Cells a Pep Talk with Light

So, what is this "magic light"? You might have heard it called Low-Level Light Therapy (LLLT). Picture it as a targeted spa day for your cells. Using very specific, low-energy wavelengths of red and near-infrared light (the same gentle spectrum found in a sunrise or sunset), PBM gives your cells the encouragement they need to work more efficiently.

Here's how it works: Inside every cell in your body are tiny engines called mitochondria. They are responsible for producing the energy, known as ATP, that fuels every single thing your body does. PBM is like a supercharger for these engines. A specific enzyme in the mitochondria, called cytochrome c oxidase, acts like a solar panel. When it soaks up the PBM light, it kicks your cellular engines into high gear.

This energy boost triggers a cascade of amazing effects:

More Cellular Fuel: With an abundance of ATP, cells have more energy to repair, regenerate, and remodel—the very essence of orthodontic treatment.

Improved Blood Flow: The light prompts the release of nitric oxide, a fantastic molecule that relaxes blood vessels. This "opens up the highways," allowing more oxygen-rich blood and vital nutrients to flood the area around your teeth, creating the perfect environment for change.

Reduced Stress: PBM helps balance the cellular environment, reducing the oxidative stress that can slow down healing.

In short, PBM isn't forcing anything. It's simply switching on your body's own natural, high-performance healing and remodeling systems.

The Science of the Shift: Moving Teeth with Ease

Orthodontic treatment is a biological dance of bone remodeling. As your braces or aligners apply gentle pressure, they signal specialized "demolition" cells (osteoclasts) to clear away bone on one side of the tooth root, making space for it to move. Simultaneously, "construction" cells (osteoblasts) get to work building new bone on the other side, securing the tooth in its new home.

PBM acts like the foreman of this microscopic construction site, ensuring the whole process runs smoothly and ahead of schedule. By energizing both the demo and construction crews, PBM helps this remodeling cycle happen much faster.

Furthermore, it promotes the growth of new blood vessels—a process called angiogenesis. The tissue around your tooth roots, the periodontal ligament, is working overtime during treatment. A rich blood supply is crucial to keep it nourished and healthy. PBM ensures this vital supply chain is robust and efficient, supporting the intense work of moving teeth.

More Than Just Speed: The Unexpected Perks

Perhaps the most celebrated part of PBM isn't just the accelerated timeline, but the profound impact it has on the patient experience.

Turning Down the Pain Dial: Anyone who has had their braces tightened knows the ache that follows. This pain is caused by inflammation. PBM is a powerful anti-inflammatory. It calms this response, significantly reducing the pain and discomfort associated with adjustments. Imagine getting through your treatment with far less reliance on painkillers. For many, this is the single greatest benefit.

Protecting Your Roots: A potential, though often minor, side effect of orthodontics is the slight shortening of tooth roots, called root resorption. It's a concern for orthodontists and patients alike. Exciting research suggests that PBM may act as a protective shield. By creating a healthier, less inflammatory environment, it helps safeguard the roots, potentially reducing this risk. Faster and safer? That's a win-win.

What Does It Look Like in Real Life?

Bringing this technology into your daily routine couldn't be simpler. PBM devices for orthodontics are typically lightweight, portable mouthpieces that you use at home. Lined with tiny, cool-to-the-touch LEDs, you simply pop the device in for a few minutes each day. It's a quick, painless session you can do while watching TV or scrolling through your phone. This ease of use is a key reason why patients love it and stick with it.

A Brighter Future for Your Smile

The journey to a perfect smile is a marathon, but Photobiomodulation offers a chance to pick up the pace and enjoy the scenery along the way. By optimizing your own biology with the gentle power of light, it promises an orthodontic experience that is not only shorter but also dramatically more comfortable.

While researchers continue to fine-tune the perfect protocols, the evidence is clear: PBM is a safe, effective, and empowering tool. It represents a shift in philosophy—from simply pushing teeth to creating the ideal biological environment for them to move. It's a future where achieving your dream smile is a faster, gentler, and all-around better experience. And that's a future worth smiling about.

The Orthodontist as Navigator: A Guide to the Hype and Hope of Faster Smiles

In the world of orthodontics, one question echoes louder than any other, whispered from the chair by patients young and old: "Are we there yet?"

This universal desire for a shorter journey to a perfect smile has created a booming industry of "shortcuts"—orthodontic acceleration techniques. They arrive in glossy brochures and slick presentations, promising to slash treatment times and revolutionize our practices. But as clinicians, we are not salespeople. We are navigators. Our job is to look past the siren song of marketing and consult the real map: the one drawn by scientific evidence. We must ask the tough questions: Does this path truly lead to the destination faster? And what is the cost of the journey?

The Gentle Glow: Is Photobiomodulation a True Shortcut?

Imagine giving your patient a high-tech compass, a device that, with a gentle, low-level light, promises to guide their teeth to their final positions more quickly. This is the allure of photobiomodulation (PBM). The collective wisdom of many studies—our trail reviews, so to speak—suggests this compass can indeed work.

But here's the crucial detail that's often lost in the excitement: not all compasses are created equal, and they don't work by just being in your pocket. The effectiveness of PBM is exquisitely sensitive. Think of it as dialing in a specific radio frequency to get a clear signal. The research points to a very specific channel for success:

The Wavelength: A near-infrared light, around 830 ± 20 nm, seems to be the sweet spot, able to penetrate the landscape of the gums and bone.

The Power: It needs enough energy to be heard. An energy density of at least 5 J/cm^2 per point is the minimum volume required to wake up the cells and get them moving.

The Consistency: This isn't a tool you use once and forget. The most promising results come from consistent, dedicated use—either daily or every other day.

If any of these parameters are off, the signal is lost. The compass spins uselessly. This explains the frustrating static in the research, where some studies report fantastic results and others hear nothing at all.

And this brings us to the most human question: even when it works perfectly, what does it mean for the traveler? A "statistically significant" result might mean saving three weeks on a two-year expedition. As their trusted guide, we must ask our patients: Is that small time savings worth the daily commitment and financial cost of this high-tech tool? For some, absolutely. For others, it's a price not worth paying.

Forging a New Path: The Surgical Detour of MOPs and Piezocision

Now, let's consider a more dramatic approach. Instead of a compass, surgical techniques like Micro-Osteoperforations (MOPs) and Piezocision are akin to actively reshaping the terrain. By creating tiny, localized disturbances in the bone, we're essentially summoning a "construction crew"—the body's own inflammatory response—to rapidly remodel the area and clear a path for the teeth to move.

The effect can be impressive. These techniques often create an immediate, noticeable burst of speed. You've successfully blasted through a rocky patch on the trail, and for a while, the pace is exhilarating.

But the evidence urges a wider view. Does that initial sprint actually shorten the entire marathon? Often, this surge is temporary. After the initial flurry of activity, the pace can slow back to normal, and the total time saved over the entire treatment journey may be less dramatic than that first burst of speed suggests.

As guides, we have a duty to describe this path honestly. It involves a surgical procedure, however "minimally invasive." This means discussing the realities of the journey: the potential for discomfort, the cost, the healing process, and the risks involved. While generally well-tolerated, we're asking our patients to take a more rugged, physically demanding detour. Is that initial burst of speed worth the climb?

The Navigator's Stance: A Conversation, Not a Prescription

The true art of modern orthodontics lies in navigating these choices with our patients, not for them. It's about spreading out the map on the table and having an honest conversation.

"Here is the traditional path," we might say. "It's reliable, it's tested, and we know exactly how long it takes. Now, here are some other options. This one involves using a special light therapy every day. It could shorten our journey by 15-30%, but it requires your diligent participation. This other path is a bit more rugged at the start; it involves a small procedure that will get things moving very quickly at first, but the overall time saved might be modest. Which journey feels right for you?"

This is the heart of informed consent. It's about translating the complex language of scientific studies into a human conversation about trade-offs. It's about managing expectations, not selling miracles.

Our ultimate destination is not just a corrected bite and a beautiful smile. It's getting our patient to that endpoint safely, comfortably, and feeling like a respected partner in their own journey. By grounding our recommendations in solid evidence and deep empathy, we move beyond the hype. We become the trusted navigators our patients deserve, guiding them wisely to a destination that is truly worth the journey.

Miniscrew-Assisted Orthodontics: Biomechanical Principles for Complex Movements

The Tiny Titan: How a Little Screw Became the Unsung Hero of Your Smile

Imagine an orchestra without a conductor, or a skyscraper built on sand. For years, orthodontists faced a similar challenge. They had the instruments to create beautiful smiles—the brackets, the wires, the bands—but sometimes, they lacked a perfectly stable, unmoving anchor to pull against. Moving one tooth often meant unintentionally nudging another. It was a delicate, frustrating dance of push-and-pull.

Then, a tiny hero arrived on the scene: the orthodontic miniscrew, or Temporary Anchorage Device (TAD). Don't let the name fool you. This isn't something you'd find at a hardware store. It's a marvel of micro-engineering, a tiny titan that has quietly revolutionized the art of building a perfect smile. It acts as a fixed point, a temporary anchor drilled into the bone, giving your orthodontist the ultimate control to achieve movements once thought impossible.

An Architect's Dream in Miniature

Think of your orthodontist as a biomechanical architect, and the miniscrew as their most advanced tool. Every millimeter of its design is a testament to form following function.

The Command Center (The Head): Peeking just above the gumline is the head, the screw's "working end." It's not a simple flat top. It's a beautifully sculpted hub of connection points—a slot here, an eyelet there—designed to be the perfect dock for the engines of tooth movement. This is where your orthodontist will loop a tiny spring to close a gap, or hook a delicate elastic chain to guide a stubborn tooth into place. The head is engineered to be strong enough to guide a tooth, yet smooth and low-profile enough that you'll barely notice it's there.

The Diplomat (The Transmucosal Neck): This is the polished, elegant collar that passes through the gum tissue, connecting the world outside with the foundation within. Its role is one of peacekeeper. Its ultrasmooth surface is designed to befriend the sensitive gum tissue, preventing irritation and discouraging plaque from setting up camp. A happy, healthy gum will form a tight seal around this collar, protecting the bone beneath and keeping the entire structure secure.

The Foundation (The Threaded Body): This is where the magic happens. The body of the screw is a helix of razor-sharp threads designed to bite into the bone with unshakeable resolve. When your orthodontist places the screw, these threads engage the bone, creating what's known as "primary stability." It's the same principle as a rock climber setting an anchor into a cliff face. The design of these threads is a science in itself, varying in depth and pitch to perfectly match the density of the bone at the chosen site, ensuring the screw stays put throughout its mission.

The Secret Ingredient: A Treaty with Your Body

The material chosen for these tiny titans is no accident. They are forged from a specific biocompatible titanium alloy, often Ti-6Al-4V. This isn't just metal; it's a material that has learned how to speak the body's language.

"Biocompatible" means your body doesn't see it as a hostile invader. It doesn't trigger an immune system alarm or cause inflammation. It simply accepts the titanium, making a peace treaty that allows it to exist in harmony with living tissue.

But titanium holds an even deeper secret: osseointegration. This is a biological superpower where living bone cells don't just tolerate the titanium; they actively grow onto and fuse with its surface. Over weeks, the bone gives the miniscrew a living embrace, locking it into place with a bond that is both structural and biological. Some miniscrews even have microscopically roughened surfaces, like a textured handshake, inviting the bone cells to grab on even tighter. This fusion of metal and living bone creates an anchor of incredible strength and stability.

The Art of Placement: A GPS for Your Jaw

Placing a miniscrew is a delicate dance of art and science, a procedure defined by precision.

First, your orthodontist becomes a cartographer of your anatomy. Using the gold standard of modern imaging—a Cone Beam Computed Tomography (CBCT) scan—they get a breathtaking 3D view of your jaw. This isn't just an X-ray; it's a high-resolution GPS map. They can see the exact thickness of your bone, trace the path of nerves and blood vessels, and measure the space between tooth roots down to a fraction of a millimeter.

With this map, they plan the mission. They might choose a spot cleverly tucked between the roots of two teeth for direct action, or anchor high on the infrazygomatic crest (cheekbone area) for its incredibly dense bone, perfect for moving a whole section of teeth. Another prime location is the hard palate, the roof of your mouth, which offers a vast, stable foundation far from any tooth roots.

The insertion itself is surprisingly gentle. After numbing the area, the orthodontist will choose their tool. For areas with softer bone, they might use a self-drilling screw, whose sharp tip elegantly carves its own path. In very dense, hard bone, they'll take a more measured approach, first creating a tiny pilot hole with a specialized drill before placing a self-tapping screw, ensuring a precise fit with minimal force.

The moment of placement is one of tactile artistry. The orthodontist feels for the subtle resistance as the threads engage, a signal that the tiny titan has found its secure home. In many cases, it can be put to work immediately, a testament to its ingenious design.

While the most common complication is a simple loosening, meticulous planning has made significant issues rare. The miniscrew is a temporary guest; once its job is done, it is removed in a simple procedure, leaving the bone to heal as if it were never there.

This tiny screw is more than just a piece of metal. It is a key that has unlocked a new level of orthodontic artistry, empowering specialists to create healthier, more confident, and more beautiful smiles with a precision and control that was once pure science fiction. It is the tiny, unsung hero, working silently within the bone to help orchestrate your perfect smile.

The Soloist and the Symphony: A New Vision of Orthodontic Power

A smile is a story. It's the first line of our personal introduction, a curve of confidence that can change a room. But crafting that story, guiding each character—each tooth—to its perfect place, is an art form built on the quiet, unyielding laws of physics. For years, orthodontists were like conductors leading a talented but unruly orchestra, where every push on one instrument created a pull on another. Moving one tooth meant risking the drift of its neighbors. It was a constant negotiation of forces, a delicate balance of reciprocal push-and-pull.

Then, everything changed. The arrival of Temporary Anchorage Devices, or TADs, was like giving our conductor a set of unmovable pillars within the stage itself. These tiny, biocompatible screws, placed directly into the bone, offered a point of absolute stability—a concept we call skeletal anchorage. Finally, the orchestra could be led with perfect precision. But how to use this newfound power? This is where the artistry truly begins, in a fundamental choice between two profound philosophies: the path of the soloist, and the way of the symphony.

The Soloist: A Private Conversation Between Anchor and Tooth

Imagine a single dancer on a vast, empty stage, tethered by a single, invisible wire to a hook in the sky. Every movement is pure, every leap and turn dictated solely by the pull of that wire. There is no one to bump into, no one to lean on. This is the soul of direct anchorage.

It is the most beautifully straightforward expression of orthodontic force. The TAD is the skyhook, the unshakeable point in the universe of the mouth. From this silent, steadfast anchor, a tiny spring or elastic chain reaches out and engages a single tooth, or perhaps a small, select group. It's a private conversation. The TAD whispers a command—"come this way"—and the tooth has no choice but to listen.

Think of a canine tooth that needs to be guided back into a space. With direct anchorage, the TAD is placed nearby, and the force is applied directly from the screw to the tooth. The anchor is the TAD; the TAD is the anchor. There are no middlemen, no unwilling participants. The immense reactive force that would normally strain the back molars, tempting them to drift forward and spoil the plan, is instead absorbed entirely by the bone. It vanishes without a trace.

This approach is a masterclass in focus and control. It's the method of choice for the purist, for the situation demanding a singular, perfect movement. Intruding a tooth that has erupted too far, closing a stubborn gap without disturbing the rest of the arch, or pulling an impacted tooth into its rightful place—these are the solos, the breathtaking moments of precision made possible by a direct, uncompromised line of force.

The Symphony: The Art of Building an Unshakeable Alliance

If direct anchorage is a solo, indirect anchorage is a full symphony. It is a more complex and subtle strategy, a masterpiece of reinforcement and shared strength. Here, the TAD doesn't take center stage as the direct mover of teeth. Instead, it plays the role of the silent benefactor, the unseen foundation that elevates an entire section of the orchestra.

In this philosophy, the orthodontist doesn't attach the force directly from the TAD to the teeth being moved. Instead, they first use the TAD to make another tooth—typically a large, sturdy molar—absolutely immovable. A rigid wire or a bonded brace acts like a declaration, lashing the molar to the TAD. It's like deputizing a citizen.

That molar, once just another tooth susceptible to unwanted reciprocal drift, is transformed. Bolstered by the TAD's skeletal stability, it becomes a pillar of the community, an anchor of absolute, unwavering strength.

Now, the real work can begin. With this newly invincible molar as a base of operations, the orthodontist can confidently apply forces to retract the front teeth, realign an entire segment, or shift the whole arch. The reactive forces crash against the reinforced molar like waves against a granite sea wall, dissipating harmlessly. The TAD, through its quiet alliance, lends its superpower of immovability to its dental partner, allowing that partner to command the movement of others without flinching.

This is the strategy for the grand movements, the sweeping changes that redefine a smile. When an entire group of front teeth needs to be brought back in unison, or a whole quadrant of teeth needs to be shifted to make space, indirect anchorage provides the robust, widespread stability required. It's not about a single line of force; it's about creating an entire zone of unyielding stability from which to conduct the beautiful, complex symphony of tooth movement.

The Artist's Choice: A Palette of Predictability

The choice between the soloist and the symphony is never arbitrary. It is a profound strategic decision based on the unique story of each patient's smile. It's about understanding the deep narrative of the forces at play.

Direct anchorage offers a clean, predictable force system. The movement is pure, the side effects minimal. It's the scalpel for a precise incision. The challenge lies in the placement—the skyhook must be positioned perfectly so that its pull creates the exact movement desired.

Indirect anchorage creates a more intricate, layered system of forces. It's the master architect's plan, reinforcing the structure before applying the load. It offers incredible flexibility, allowing the orthodontist to create a custom anchor unit tailored to the grandest of treatment plans. The challenge is ensuring the connection between the TAD and its dental deputy is perfectly rigid, a flawless fusion of power.

Ultimately, these two philosophies are not rivals, but partners in the modern orthodontist's toolkit. They represent a mastery over the physics of tooth movement that was once unimaginable. By choosing the path of the soloist for a moment of focused perfection, or the way of the symphony for a powerful, sweeping transformation, the orthodontist steps beyond the role of a technician and becomes a true artist—a sculptor of confidence, a choreographer of smiles, and the storyteller who gives every tooth its perfect place in the narrative of a beautiful life.

The Architect's Anchor: How a Tiny Screw Revolutionized the Art of the Smile

For the longest time, orthodontics operated under a fundamental law of physics, as frustrating as it was unyielding: for every action, there is an equal and opposite reaction. Imagine an orthodontist as an architect, trying to perfect the delicate archway of a smile. Every time they pushed a stray tooth into place, another, somewhere else, would push back. Straightening a smile was a constant negotiation, a balancing act of compromises. To prevent the entire structure from shifting undesirably, they often resorted to clumsy, external scaffolding—unwieldy headgear that turned the patient's cooperation into the most critical, and often weakest, link in the entire process.

Then, almost silently, a revolution arrived. It wasn't a flashy new machine or a radical theory, but something impossibly small and brilliantly simple: the Temporary Anchorage Device, or TAD.

These tiny, biocompatible screws are the orthodontic equivalent of finding bedrock. Placed strategically into the bone, they act as an immovable anchor, a point of absolute stability that finally breaks the old rule of action-and-reaction. They don't push back. They simply hold their ground. This "absolute anchorage" has given orthodontists the power of a sculptor's steady hand, allowing them to move teeth with a precision that was once the stuff of dreams. They've transformed the craft, turning once-impossible challenges into routine artistry.

Lowering the Foundation: Solving the Open Bite

Picture a smile that doesn't quite meet in the front, leaving a persistent gap. This is an anterior open bite, and often, the culprits are the back molars. Having grown too far down, they act like a fulcrum, propping the jaw open and preventing the front teeth from ever coming together. For an orthodontist, pushing those over-erupted molars back up into the jawbone—a movement called intrusion—was like trying to push a piling back into the earth without disturbing the surrounding landscape. The force required would almost always make other teeth shift in protest.

This is where the magic of the TAD becomes crystal clear. An orthodontist can now place a tiny TAD in the bone just above these tall molars. A gentle, continuous force, applied with a simple elastic chain, then coaxes the molars upward, back into the jaw. It's a quiet, targeted pressure with a dramatic result. As the molars intrude, the entire jaw can pivot slightly upward and forward, like a drawbridge gracefully closing. The open bite vanishes, and in the process, the patient's entire facial profile can soften, transforming a "long face" appearance into one of natural balance. It's a non-surgical facelift, achieved with nothing more than a tiny anchor and a deep understanding of facial architecture.

Redrawing the Blueprint: Perfecting the Profile

Many smiles need space. To relieve crowding or pull back a protrusive profile, orthodontists often need to remove a pair of premolar teeth. This creates a valuable gap, but using that space wisely was historically a challenge. The goal is to pull the six front teeth backward as a single, solid unit. But as you pulled them back, the anchor teeth in the back would inevitably slide forward, stealing precious real estate. It was like trying to pull a curtain closed, only to have the curtain rod shrink at the same time.

TADs have completely rewritten this process. By placing an anchor in the back of the mouth—a steadfast, unyielding point—the orthodontist can attach a line directly to the front teeth and pull. The front teeth glide backward into their new home, and the molars don't move an inch. The entire extraction space is used exactly as intended. This "en-masse retraction" is not only incredibly efficient and predictable, but it also completely untethers the outcome from a patient's need to wear headgear. It simplifies the most complex phase of treatment into a beautifully straightforward maneuver.

Expanding the Floor Plan: Making Space Without Demolition

Sometimes, the entire upper row of teeth is too far forward, creating an overjet. The traditional solution was often to push all the upper molars backward—a movement called distalization—to create space. But this relied almost entirely on the patient diligently wearing their headgear. If they didn't, the treatment would stall.

TADs offer a brilliant workaround that feels more like smart design than brute force. By placing an anchor in the roof of the mouth or on the cheek-side of the jaw, an orthodontist can use it as a winch point. Springs or elastics run from this fixed point directly to the molars, pulling them backward with a steady, reliable force that works 24/7, no patient compliance required. Because the anchor is absolute, there's no reciprocal force pushing the front teeth forward. It's pure, controlled movement that can often eliminate the need for extractions altogether—a non-invasive way to expand the floor plan of the smile.

The Art of Asymmetry: The Final, Perfecting Touch

No face is perfectly symmetrical, and neither is any smile. A dental midline can be shifted to one side, or a bite can be off-kilter unilaterally. Trying to fix one side of the mouth with traditional braces was like trying to paint one half of a room without getting a single drop on the other half. The forces were shared across the arch, making a truly one-sided fix nearly impossible.

TADs, however, allow for masterpiece-level detailing. Because they are independent anchors, they let an orthodontist apply force with laser-like precision. Is the midline off to the right? Place a TAD on the right side and gently pull that segment of teeth back into alignment, while the left side remains completely untouched. Is a single molar out of place? Intrude, rotate, or move it with a force that is unique to that tooth alone. This ability to isolate movement gives orthodontists the freedom to correct asymmetries with an elegance and predictability that was previously out of reach.

Ultimately, TADs have done more than just introduce a new tool. They have fundamentally changed the conversation between the orthodontist and the patient. Cases once deemed too complex, or that would have required invasive surgery, are now confidently treated in the orthodontist's chair. The reliance on headgear is fading, and treatment times are often shorter and more predictable. By providing a point of absolute stability, these tiny anchors have given orthodontists the freedom to be true architects of the smile, sculpting with a level of control and artistry that brings life-changing results to their patients.

Your Smile's Secret Weapon: The Unlikely Alliance That's Changing Orthodontics

We all know the star of the show: clear aligners. They're the rockstars of the orthodontic world, the sleek, nearly invisible solution that lets you straighten your teeth without the whole world knowing. They're brilliant, convenient, and have made millions of people fall in love with their smiles again.

But even a rockstar needs a world-class roadie—that unsung hero working behind the scenes to make sure the show goes off without a hitch.

For clear aligners, that hero is a tiny but mighty ally called a TAD, or Temporary Anchorage Device. On their own, both are impressive. But together? They create a partnership so powerful it's redefining what's possible, turning even the most complex orthodontic challenges into stunning success stories. This isn't just about straightening teeth; it's about unlocking the full potential of your smile.

The A-Lister: Understanding Clear Aligners

Think of your clear aligners as your smile's personal choreographer. Each tray is a meticulously planned dance step, guiding your teeth with a gentle, persistent nudge toward their grand finale. They excel at the elegant, sweeping movements—closing small gaps, untangling minor crowding, and orchestrating many common smile makeovers.

Their charm is obvious. You can pop them out for a coffee date or a family photo, and they work their magic with such subtlety that most people won't even notice they're there.

But every star has their limits. Aligners work by pushing off of your other teeth. It's like trying to push a heavy piece of furniture across a shag carpet—you might move the furniture, but you'll probably bunch up the carpet, too. For some really tough jobs, like moving a stubborn back tooth way back or pulling a tooth down into place, the aligner needs more than just your other teeth to push against. It needs an immovable object. It needs a solid wall.

The Unsung Hero: What on Earth is a TAD?

Enter the TAD, the secret weapon in your orthodontist's toolkit. Forget the clinical-sounding name for a moment. A TAD is simply a tiny, biocompatible titanium anchor, about the size of a stud in an earring. It's placed temporarily and painlessly into your jawbone during a quick visit.

The TAD's superpower is its stillness. It's the ultimate anchor. While your teeth are meant to move, a TAD provides a fixed, unbudging point to pull or push from. It's the solid wall in our furniture-moving analogy. There's no "reciprocal movement," no unwanted shifting of other teeth. It's pure, focused force, directed with GPS-level accuracy right where it needs to go.

And the "temporary" part is key. Once its mission is complete, it's removed, leaving no trace behind. It was just there to help out during the toughest parts of the journey.

The Dream Team: When Aligner Grace Meets TAD Power

This is where the magic happens. The aligner continues to be the overall director of your treatment, managing the big picture and keeping your teeth on their prescribed path. But for those "boss-level" challenges? We call in the TAD.

Here are a few of the missions this dynamic duo can accomplish:

Operation Gummy Smile Correction (Intrusion): Have you ever wished your upper front teeth were just a little shorter for a more balanced smile? Moving teeth up into the jawbone is incredibly difficult for aligners alone. But with a TAD placed discreetly above those teeth, a tiny elastic can provide a gentle, direct upward pull. The TAD does the heavy lifting, while the aligner ensures the teeth move perfectly as a unit.

The Great Molar Migration (Distalization): Let's say you need to move your back molars backward to create more room for crowded front teeth. It's one of the toughest moves in orthodontics. Using just aligners is like trying to push a car from the backseat—you'll probably just push yourself back into the seat. By placing TADs at the back of your mouth, we can create a direct line of force to pull those molars back, without the front teeth budging an inch forward. It's the difference between hoping and knowing the movement will be perfect.

Bringing a Shy Tooth to the Party (Extrusion): Sometimes, a tooth hasn't fully emerged and needs to be gently guided down into its proper place. A TAD can provide the perfect, steady anchor point to coax the tooth into the smile line, while the aligner ensures it lands in the exact right spot.

The Real-World Wins

For you, the patient, this partnership is a game-changer.

Predictability You Can Count On: It takes the guesswork out of complex movements. Your orthodontist can plan with incredible precision, leading to more reliable and beautiful results.

Often, a Faster Finish Line: By tackling the hardest movements with greater efficiency, TADs can frequently shorten your overall treatment time. You get to your dream smile sooner.

Opening the Door for More People: Many cases once considered "too complicated" for clear aligners are now perfectly treatable. This means more people can enjoy the aesthetic, comfortable experience of aligner therapy.

Worried about the TAD itself? Don't be. The placement is quick, done with local anesthetic, and most patients report little more than a day of mild soreness. It's a tiny step that delivers a giant leap forward in your treatment.

A New Era for Your Smile

The fusion of TADs and clear aligners is more than just a technique; it's a philosophy. It's about combining the art of aesthetics with the science of biomechanics. It's about giving you the discreet, comfortable treatment you want, with the powerful, predictable results you deserve.

So if you've been told your case is too complex for clear aligners, it might be time for a second opinion. The superhero sidekick your aligners have been waiting for is here, and together, they're ready to build you the smile you've always imagined.

Part IV: The Expanding Role of the Orthodontist in Interdisciplinary Care

Airway-Focused Orthodontics: Diagnosis and Management of Sleep-Disordered Breathing

Your Face is Telling a Story. Are You Listening?

Forget for a moment that your airway is a tube. Instead, picture it as a delicate, living river, its path sculpted by the very landscape of your face. This river of breath is not housed in a static tunnel of bone and flesh; it flows through a dynamic, ever-changing valley shaped by your jaws, your tongue, and the intricate architecture of your skull. Its journey can be wide and effortless, or it can be a struggle through a narrow, crowded gorge. This is the story your face tells, and an orthodontist might just be the one who knows how to read it.

The Architecture of a Breath

Every breath you take is shaped by the house it lives in—your craniofacial structure. If the foundation is small or poorly aligned, the entire house feels cramped. This is especially true while you sleep, when the world goes quiet and your body is supposed to be rebuilding.

Think of your upper jaw, the maxilla, as the ceiling of your mouth and the floor of your nasal passages. When this ceiling is narrow and vaulted, it crowds the very space you need to breathe through your nose. Air struggles to get through, like trying to navigate a cramped attic. This is why so many people become mouth-breathers. It's a detour, a less efficient back road your body takes out of necessity. But this detour comes with a cost: a dry mouth, a vulnerable throat, and over time, it can even guide a child's face to grow downward instead of forward, compounding the problem.

Now, look to the lower jaw, the mandible. This is the foundation for your tongue, that powerful, restless muscle. If the mandible is small or sits too far back, it's like having a living room that's too small for its furniture. The tongue has nowhere to go. During the day, you subconsciously hold it in place. But at night, when your muscles surrender to sleep, the tongue falls back, trespassing into the precious, shared space of your throat.

This nightly intrusion is the muffled drumbeat of a snore. When it blocks the river of breath entirely, it becomes the silent, startling pause of obstructive sleep apnea (OSA).

The Thief in the Night

Obstructive sleep apnea is more than just bad snoring. It's a thief that steals your rest, moment by moment. Each time your airway collapses, your brain sends out a panic signal, jolting you just awake enough to gasp for air. You may not remember these dozens, or even hundreds, of nightly interruptions, but your body does.

You feel it in the morning fog that won't lift, the persistent fatigue that coffee can't touch. You see it in the dark circles under your eyes. But the unseen consequences are far more sinister: high blood pressure, heart disease, diabetes, and a constant strain on your mind and mood. In children, this nightly battle for air can masquerade as ADHD, learning disabilities, or behavioral problems, as their growing brains are starved of restorative sleep.

The Orthodontist as Airway Detective

This is where the story shifts. Traditionally, we see orthodontists as smile designers, masters of alignment and aesthetics. But a new understanding is casting them in a far more vital role: as airway detectives and restorers of breath.

An orthodontist is trained to see the story of your growth. They can spot the subtle clues of a compromised airway long before it becomes a crisis. They see the recessed chin, the crowded teeth, the high, narrow palate, and they don't just see a cosmetic issue—they see a potential struggle for breath. Using advanced imaging, they can measure the exact dimensions of your airway, turning suspicion into certainty.

More Than Straight Teeth: Remodeling for Breath

Airway-focused orthodontics isn't about forcing teeth into line; it's about creating the space for them to exist in harmony with a healthy airway. It's about remodeling the very architecture of the face to free the river of breath.

For a child with a narrow upper jaw, a palatal expander can gently widen the bone. This is a profound change. As the maxilla expands, the floor of the nasal cavity widens with it, opening up the primary airway. It's like raising the ceiling in that cramped attic, allowing for the effortless, healthy flow of nasal breathing.

For a lower jaw that's set back, specialized appliances can guide its growth forward, creating a proper home for the tongue. In adults, a custom mandibular advancement device (MAD) worn at night can act as a gentle brace, holding the jaw forward and preventing the tongue from collapsing into the throat. It's a simple, elegant solution that keeps the airway open all night long.

This philosophy avoids the old-school approach of pulling teeth to make room. Instead of shrinking the dental arches, the goal is to develop them forward and outward, creating a beautiful smile as a natural consequence of creating a healthy, spacious foundation.

A Symphony of Health

This work is not done in a silo. An airway-focused orthodontist is part of a collaborative team—a symphony of specialists dedicated to your well-being. They work with sleep doctors who diagnose the disorder, ENT specialists who check for obstructions like tonsils, and myofunctional therapists who retrain the muscles of the face and tongue to function properly.

This is the future of orthodontics, a holistic vision where a beautiful smile is the outward sign of a deeper, more fundamental wellness. It's the recognition that the way we breathe is the way we live, and that sometimes, the path to a healthier, more vibrant life begins by reshaping the landscape of the face to finally let the river flow free.

Beyond the Brace: How Your Orthodontist Became an Unexpected Guardian of Your Sleep

We've all known that feeling. Waking up after eight hours in bed feeling like you've barely slept a wink. The bone-deep exhaustion that a third cup of coffee can't touch. For our kids, it might look like trouble focusing in class or unexplained irritability. We chalk it up to stress, aging, or just a part of life. But what if the first clue to solving this profound mystery of fatigue wasn't in a doctor's office or a sleep lab, but in the orthodontist's chair?

The role of the orthodontist is undergoing a quiet revolution. For generations, we've seen them as the architects of the perfect smile, masters of wires and brackets who straighten teeth for a picture-perfect grin. But today, they are looking past the pearly gates of our teeth and into a far more critical space: the hidden, vital airway that gives us life while we sleep. They are becoming the frontline detectives in the case against a silent thief: sleep-disordered breathing (SDB).

The Unseen Chokehold

Imagine, night after night, trying to breathe through a pinched straw. This is the harrowing reality of obstructive sleep apnea (OSA), the most common form of SDB. As you sleep, the airway collapses, cutting off oxygen to your brain and body in a repeated, silent chokehold. It's far more than just snoring. It's a nightly battle for air that leaves you physically and mentally drained.

This nightly struggle is a thief that steals more than just rest. In children, it can rob them of their growth, their focus at school, and their emotional stability, often masquerading as ADHD or behavioral problems. In adults, the stakes are even higher, dramatically increasing the risk of heart attacks, strokes, high blood pressure, and diabetes. It steals our energy, our joy, and our ability to be present in our own lives.

The New Chairside Investigation

The modern orthodontist has become a keen-eyed detective, and their investigation begins with a simple conversation. The questions may seem routine, but they're digging for clues: "Do you snore? Is it loud enough to bother your partner? Do you ever wake up gasping? Do you feel truly refreshed in the morning?" For parents, the questions are different: "Does your child wet the bed? Do they have night terrors? Are they a restless sleeper?"

These questions open the door to the physical examination, where the orthodontist dusts for fingerprints of an airway struggle. They see things we would never notice:

A Scalloped Tongue: Wavy indentations along the sides of the tongue are the tell-tale marks left by it pressing against the teeth. It's a fingerprint proving the tongue is fighting for space in a crowded airway.

The Silent Alarm of Mouth Breathing: Chronic mouth breathing isn't just a habit; it's a red flag that breathing through the nose is compromised, affecting everything from facial development to gum health.

A Glimpse of the Blockade: A quick look in the mouth can reveal enlarged tonsils—like two bouncers blocking the entrance to a vital club.

The Architectural Clues: A high, narrow roof of the mouth (palate) or a small, recessed lower jaw are architectural flaws in our facial structure that can force the tongue backward, obstructing the path of air. Even teeth grinding (bruxism) can be a sign of the body struggling to open the airway during sleep.

The Blueprint for Breath

A detective's hunch is powerful, but modern cases are solved with technology. The game-changer in orthodontics is Cone Beam Computed Tomography (CBCT). This isn't your old, flat dental X-ray. A CBCT scan creates a stunning 3D blueprint of your skull, jaws, and most importantly, your pharyngeal airway. Your orthodontist can digitally fly through this map of your throat, measuring its width and pinpointing the exact location of a potential bottleneck.

But this blueprint has one limitation: it's a static photograph taken while you're awake. It doesn't show what happens when the lights go out and your muscles relax. It doesn't capture the crime in progress.

That's where the future, arriving now in 2025 and beyond, gets truly exciting. Imagine having CCTV footage of the airway itself. Technologies like Swept-Source Optical Coherence Tomography (OCT) are on the horizon, promising ultra-high-resolution, dynamic imaging that could one day show the airway collapsing in real-time. Paired with Artificial Intelligence (AI) acting as a super-powered forensic analyst, these tools will be able to spot risks with breathtaking speed and accuracy.

Assembling the Task Force

Let's be clear: your orthodontist isn't the one who will officially diagnose you with sleep apnea. That crucial role belongs to a sleep physician, who uses a comprehensive overnight sleep study (polysomnogram) to get the final verdict.

Instead, the orthodontist is the one who sounds the alarm. They are the crucial first responder who sees the anatomical evidence and recognizes the danger. They are the ones who assemble the task force—connecting you with sleep physicians, ENTs, and other specialists who can solve the case. By identifying the risk early, they initiate a life-changing journey toward diagnosis and treatment. In some cases, especially for growing children, orthodontic treatment itself can help guide facial development to create a healthier, more open airway for life.

This is more than a new trend; it's a profound shift toward holistic health. It's a commitment to understanding that the alignment of a jaw can impact the quality of a life. By looking beyond the smile and into the airway, orthodontists are not just straightening teeth. They are safeguarding our breath, restoring our energy, and protecting our very well-being. They are ensuring the path to a beautiful smile is also the path to a healthier life.

Beyond the Smile: The Hidden World of Airway Orthodontics

We've all been taught to think of orthodontics as a journey toward a perfect smile—a straight, beautiful alignment of teeth that builds confidence. But what if that was only half the story? What if the true masterpiece wasn't just the smile, but the silent, life-giving river of air that flows behind it?

Welcome to the world of airway-focused orthodontics, a field that sees beyond the teeth and into the very architecture of our breath. It understands a profound truth: the shape of our jaws, the curve of our palate, and the position of our chin are the invisible blueprints that determine how we breathe, how we sleep, and ultimately, how we live.

A constricted airway is like trying to draw life through a pinched straw. It's the stuffy, restless night, the chronic mouth breathing that dries the lips, the persistent fatigue that clouds the day. It's the child who struggles to focus in class, or the adult whose snoring is a nightly cry for more air. For years, we saw these as isolated problems. Now, we see the common thread: a structural bottleneck in the airway.

And this is where the modern orthodontist becomes less of a tooth-straightener and more of an architect of breath, using incredible tools to widen the channels and set the flow of air free.

Reshaping the Landscape: The Magic of Palatal Expansion

Imagine the upper jaw, the maxilla, as the very foundation of the mid-face. It's not just the arch that holds your upper teeth; it's also the floor of your nasal cavity. For a growing child, a narrow palate is a double jeopardy—it crowds the teeth and shrinks the airway above it, forcing them into a habit of mouth breathing.

For the Growing Child: Rapid Palatal Expansion (RPE)

In childhood, the bones of the palate are connected by a growth seam, a pliable suture full of potential. RPE is the key that unlocks this potential. It's a small, gentle device that, with a simple daily turn, applies a whisper of pressure. It doesn't push teeth; it nudges the very bones apart, encouraging the maxilla to grow to its full, intended width.

The result is a beautiful chain reaction. As the palate widens, the floor of the nasal passage expands in perfect harmony. Suddenly, the resistance is gone. Air flows easily through the nose, as nature intended. This simple act can be life-altering. It invites the tongue to rest properly on the roof of the mouth, encourages healthy facial development, and, most importantly, transforms a struggling mouth-breather into a peaceful nasal-breather. It's not just correcting a crossbite; it's laying a foundation for a lifetime of better sleep and better health.

For the Adult: A Feat of Bio-Engineering (MARPE)

What happens when that growth seam has fused, when the jaw's landscape has hardened into adult form? For decades, the only answer was invasive surgery. But innovation has brought a game-changer: Mini-implant Assisted Rapid Palatal Expansion (MARPE).

MARPE is a marvel of modern orthodontics. By anchoring the expansion device directly to the bone with tiny, temporary implants, it can achieve what was once thought impossible. The force is no longer on the teeth, but on the bone itself, allowing orthodontists to reopen that fused suture and achieve true skeletal expansion in adults.

For an adult suffering from the effects of a constricted airway—from snoring to diagnosed sleep apnea—MARPE can feel like a miracle. It's a minimally invasive way to physically create more space to breathe, reducing nasal resistance and giving the tongue the room it needs to stay out of the airway during sleep. It's a structural solution to a structural problem, offering a wider smile as a beautiful side effect of a healthier, more open airway.

Guiding the Flow: The Power of Advancing the Jaw

The airway isn't just a tunnel; it's a dynamic space influenced by the position of the jaw. A lower jaw that is set back or "recessed" can push the tongue backward, turning this large, relaxed muscle into the primary obstruction during sleep.

This is where functional appliances and Mandibular Advancement Devices (MADs) come in. Think of them as guides that gently coax the lower jaw forward into a healthier, more open posture.

In a growing child, these appliances can actually encourage forward growth of the mandible, permanently correcting the underlying issue. In adults, custom-fitted MADs, worn during sleep, hold the jaw forward, pulling the tongue with it. This single movement can be the difference between a night of choking and gasping and a night of silent, restorative sleep. It's an elegant solution that prevents the collapse of the airway, dramatically reducing snoring and treating obstructive sleep apnea for those who find CPAP machines difficult to tolerate.

A Symphony of Health

The shift to airway-focused orthodontics is a shift toward seeing the whole person. It begins with listening—asking about sleep, energy levels, and breathing habits. It's made visible through incredible technology like Cone-Beam Computed Tomography (CBCT), which gives a stunning 3D view of the airway's unique geography.

And it thrives on collaboration. The airway orthodontist often works as part of a team, consulting with ENT specialists on tonsils and sinuses, with sleep physicians on diagnoses, and with myofunctional therapists who help retrain the muscles to embrace these new, healthier postures.

The ultimate goal is to restore the body's most fundamental rhythm. By widening the palate and positioning the jaw, these treatments do more than create space for teeth—they create space for life. They help turn restless nights into deep sleep, brain fog into sharp focus, and listless fatigue into vibrant energy.

The most beautiful smile, after all, isn't just the one you can see. It's the one that comes from a body that can finally, truly, and deeply breathe.

The Unseen Thief of Sleep

Imagine a thief who visits you every night. This thief doesn't steal your valuables, but something far more precious: your breath, your energy, your very vitality. You go to bed exhausted and wake up feeling like you've run a marathon in your sleep. A fog follows you through your day, clouding your thoughts and stealing your joy. This is the lonely reality for millions living with Sleep-Disordered Breathing (SDB) and Obstructive Sleep Apnea (OSA). It's a nightly struggle that happens in the dark, a silent battle that leaves you drained.

But what if you could assemble a team of specialists—a fellowship of guardians—to not only catch this thief but to rebuild your fortress so it can never break in again? The path to reclaiming your life from the clutches of OSA isn't walked alone. It requires a trio of experts, each with a unique key to unlock the puzzle of your sleep. This isn't just a treatment plan; it's a mission to restore your breath and give you back your days.

The Night Navigator: Your Sleep Physician

The journey begins with the Sleep Physician, the master navigator of the hidden world of sleep. You might know the symptoms—the bone-rattling snores, the choking gasps your partner mentions, the relentless daytime exhaustion—but these are just whispers from a distant shore. The sleep physician is the one who charts the unknown territory.

They are the captain of the diagnostic voyage, using an incredible mapmaking tool called polysomnography (PSG). For one night, you are connected to a web of sensors that tells a secret story. It's a story written in your brainwaves, your heartbeats, the rise and fall of your chest, and the silent pauses in your breath. The PSG reveals the truth of the night, calculating your Apnea-Hypopnea Index (AHI)—a score that grades the severity of the thief's visits. Is it a petty intruder or a master burglar? This single, crucial piece of intelligence, delivered by the sleep physician, becomes the guiding star for the entire team. They are the ones who can say, "Here, this is where the map is torn. This is where the journey to healing begins."

The Gatekeeper of the Airway: Your ENT Specialist

Once the navigator has identified the problem, the next guardian is called: the ENT (Ear, Nose, and Throat) specialist. Think of them as the gatekeeper and architect of your body's most vital pathway—the airway. While the sleep study reveals the what, the ENT discovers the where. They are masters of anatomy, embarking on an expedition through the intricate landscape of your respiratory tract.

With a skilled eye and sometimes a tiny, flexible camera, they explore the nasal passages, the throat, and the hidden corners where soft tissues reside. They search for the physical culprits, the roadblocks on your road to breath. Are overgrown tonsils or adenoids acting like fallen boulders, especially in children? Is a deviated septum a wall built in the middle of a tunnel? Is a soft palate collapsing like a tent in the wind? The ENT's role is profoundly hands-on. They are the surgeons who can clear the path, performing procedures that remove these physical obstructions. They don't just treat the problem; they physically liberate your breath, ensuring the gateway for air is wide open.

The Architect of Breath: Your Orthodontist

For decades, we saw orthodontists as the artists who straightened our smiles. But their true role is far deeper. They are the Architects of Breath, with a profound understanding of the very foundation of your airway: your facial structure. They see that a beautiful smile is wonderful, but a smile that allows you to breathe freely is life-changing.

The orthodontist is often the first to see the subtle clues of a compromised airway, especially in a growing child—the tell-tale sign of mouth breathing, a high, narrow palate that cramps the nasal cavity, or a lower jaw that is set too far back, crowding the airway space. Their tools are not merely for aesthetics; they are instruments of architectural change. A rapid palatal expander doesn't just make room for teeth; it widens the entire floor of the nasal cavity, inviting in more air. A mandibular advancement device doesn't just align a bite; it gently guides the jaw and tongue forward during sleep, pulling them out of the way of the collapsing airway. They don't just rearrange the furniture; they expand the entire room.

A Masterpiece of Collaboration

Here is where the true magic unfolds. These three experts are not a relay team, passing a baton from one to the next. They are a true fellowship, working in constant dialogue, huddling over the same map.

Imagine them together: The Sleep Physician presents the navigator's chart, showing the precise moments of collapse. The ENT points to the anatomical roadblocks they've discovered—the "fallen boulders." And the Orthodontist brings the architectural blueprints of the jaw and face, showing how the very foundation might be the underlying issue.

Together, they craft a plan of attack. Perhaps the ENT first clears the immediate obstructions, like a pathfinder clearing a trail. Then, the Orthodontist begins the deeper work of reshaping the landscape, widening the path into a highway. All the while, the Sleep Physician monitors the progress, conducting follow-up studies to ensure the thief has been permanently evicted. This constant communication, this fusion of expertise, is the difference between patching a problem and rebuilding a life. It's a promise that every angle is being considered, every stone unturned, in the singular quest to let you breathe. The result is more than just a quiet night; it's the dawn of a new, more vibrant life.

The Ortho-Surgical Interface: Integrated Planning for Orthognathic Procedures

The Face in the Mirror: When a Perfect Smile Needs a Deeper Foundation

We learn to read faces before we learn to read words. We search them for comfort, for truth, for a sense of who we are. But what happens when the face you see in the mirror doesn't feel like your own? It's not about a crooked tooth or a small gap—braces, the miracle workers of modern dentistry, can beautifully handle that. This is a dissonance that runs deeper, a feeling that the very architecture of your face, the foundation of bone beneath the skin, is somehow out of sync.

Think of your smile as a masterpiece. Orthodontics is the artist, meticulously arranging every detail to perfection. But if the canvas itself—the jaw—is warped, buckled, or improperly sized, the artist's best work can only go so far. The underlying disharmony remains. This is the moment when the conversation must change, moving beyond the alignment of teeth to the very structure of you. This is the world of orthognathic surgery.

More Than a Bite: Reading the Signs in Your Own Reflection

The decision to reshape the jaw is never made lightly. It's a path chosen when the disconnect between the upper and lower jaws is so profound that it impacts daily life in ways both seen and unseen. It's for those who have reached the end of their physical growth, whose bones have settled into a final, unaccommodating position.

For some, orthodontists can perform a kind of beautiful illusion, a "camouflage," repositioning teeth to mask a minor skeletal imbalance. But for many, this is like hanging a picture to hide a crack in the wall—it doesn't fix the foundation. When the issue is severe, surgery becomes the only path to true, lasting harmony. So, what does this foundational imbalance look like?

The Jaw That Leads the Way (Severe Underbite)

You see it in profile. The lower jaw juts forward, assertive and prominent, pushing the lower teeth past the upper. This is more than a "strong chin"; it's a daily functional puzzle. Chewing becomes a challenge of shearing instead of grinding. Certain sounds in speech might carry a subtle lisp. It can create an aesthetic you never chose, a permanent bulldog expression that doesn't match the spirit within. Braces can't shorten a bone that has grown too long. Surgery is the only way to gently set the lower jaw back, allowing your bite—and your profile—to finally meet in a comfortable, natural embrace.

The Chin That Hides (Severe Overbite)

Conversely, some look in the mirror and see a chin that seems to retreat, a lower jaw overshadowed by the upper. This can create the appearance of "buck teeth," not because the teeth are necessarily at fault, but because their foundation is set too far back. This isn't just about appearance; it's about function and comfort. The upper teeth may bite down onto the sensitive gum tissue of the lower jaw, causing pain and damage. The jaw joint (TMJ) can be under constant strain, leading to chronic pain and headaches. Closing your lips can feel like a conscious effort. Jaw surgery brings the lower jaw forward, restoring balance, relieving strain, and giving the chin the place it was always meant to occupy.

The Smile That Reveals Too Much, or Hides a Secret (Vertical Issues)

A smile is a universal expression of joy, but for some, it's a source of self-consciousness. When the upper jaw is vertically too long, a full smile can reveal an excessive amount of gum tissue—the "gummy smile." Often, this goes hand-in-hand with an "open bite," where the front teeth don't touch at all. Imagine the simple frustration of being unable to bite into a slice of pizza or a crisp apple. The joy of food is diminished. Surgery can reposition the entire upper jaw, moving it upward to create a smile that showcases teeth, not gums, and closes the frustrating gap, finally allowing the front teeth to meet.

The Face in Soft Focus (Facial Asymmetry)

Perfect symmetry is a myth, a digital creation. But significant asymmetry is a tangible reality for some. It's when one side of the jaw has grown more than the other, creating a noticeable tilt or shift in your facial features. It can make you feel like you're perpetually looking at yourself in a slightly warped mirror. This imbalance can cascade into functional problems—an uneven bite, chewing difficulties, and joint pain. Jaw surgery is the only way to address this fundamental imbalance, re-centering your features to create a sense of harmony and peace.

The Architect's New Vision: AI in Rebuilding a Foundation

For decades, the path to jaw surgery was planned with X-rays, physical models, and the seasoned intuition of surgeons and orthodontists. Today, we are witnessing a revolution. Artificial intelligence is transforming this intricate process, offering a level of foresight that was once the stuff of science fiction.

Imagine creating a perfect digital twin of your own skull. AI algorithms analyze 3D scans with breathtaking precision, mapping every contour and dimension of your unique skeletal structure. This isn't just a static picture; it's a dynamic simulation. The AI can identify foundational issues with uncanny accuracy, flagging cases where orthodontics alone would be a compromise.

This digital foresight is a profound gift. It allows for honest, transparent conversations from day one, managing expectations and building trust. More importantly, it allows the surgical team to perform the entire surgery virtually, dozens of times, before ever making an incision. They can test different approaches, predict the exact outcome, and even show you a stunningly realistic preview of your new profile. This isn't just planning; it's digital rehearsal for a life-changing performance.

Finding Your Harmony

The journey of orthognathic surgery is a deep collaboration—a partnership between you, your orthodontist, and your oral surgeon. It's a commitment to a future where your smile is not just beautiful, but healthy; where your bite is not just aligned, but powerful; and where the face you see in the mirror finally feels like home. It is for those moments when polishing the details is no longer enough, and the time has come to rebuild the foundation, creating a masterpiece of function, health, and identity that will last a lifetime.

The Overture Before the Transformation: A Story of a Smile in the Making

Before a life-altering surgery can sculpt a new harmony for your face and jaw, a quiet, meticulous performance must take place. This is pre-surgical orthodontics, and it's far more than just straightening teeth. It is the art of preparing the stage, of tuning the instruments, of composing the masterpiece that your future smile will become.

Think of your body as an orchestra, one where some instruments are not quite in their right place. For years, the other musicians—your teeth—have strained to play in tune, compensating for the imbalance. They've leaned in, tilted back, and twisted themselves into new positions, all in a heroic effort to create a functional melody. This is called "compensation," and it's your body's beautiful, imperfect attempt to hide a deeper, skeletal dissonance.

But to create a true symphony, you can't just play louder. You must first retune every single instrument.

Finding Your True Note: The Courage of Decompensation

The most profound and often misunderstood movement in this process is called "decompensation." It is the brave act of undoing all the natural camouflage your teeth have created over the years.

Imagine your lower jaw is set back. To help you bite, your lower teeth have likely fanned forward, reaching desperately to meet their partners above. They are hiding the true distance between your jaws. Decompensation is the journey of guiding those teeth back to their honest, upright position on the jawbone.

Here lies the paradox that requires your trust: as your orthodontist works, your bite will likely look and feel worse. The gap you've always tried to hide will suddenly be exposed, raw and more apparent than ever. It can feel like a step backward, a moment of jarring dissonance in the music.

But this is the most crucial part of the overture. We must reveal the true, unmasked reality of the skeletal disharmony. It's like pulling back a velvet curtain to show the bare stage. Only then can the surgeon, your co-maestro in this performance, see the precise landscape they need to transform. This temporary worsening isn't a failure; it's the sound of truth, the necessary tuning before the beautiful chord can be struck.

Arranging the Orchestra: The Art of Arch Coordination

With the instruments retuned, the next movement begins: arranging the orchestra. This is "arch coordination," the art of shaping your upper and lower arches of teeth so that after surgery, they will nestle into each other in a perfect, harmonious embrace.

Imagine two intricate, beautiful gears. Separately, they are stunning. But for the machine to work, their teeth must interlock with flawless precision. Your dental arches are those gears. The goal is a "Class I occlusion"—a relationship so stable and so perfectly aligned that the forces of your bite flow through your jaw in a balanced, healthy way.

This is a three-dimensional ballet:

Width (Transverse): Like arranging the violin section to match the breadth of the cellos, your orthodontist will ensure the width of your upper arch perfectly corresponds to the lower one.

Depth (Anteroposterior): The front-to-back flow of the arches is refined, ensuring a seamless fit from your front incisors to your back molars.

Height (Vertical): The biting surfaces of your teeth are leveled to create a smooth, harmonious plane, eliminating any jarring "notes" when you chew.

Using the gentle, persistent guidance of archwires, elastics, and sometimes tiny anchors, your orthodontist is the conductor, coaxing each tooth into its final, perfect position in the orchestral pit.

A Duet of Masters: The Surgeon and the Orthodontist

This entire performance is a seamless duet between two masters: your orthodontist and your oral surgeon. They share the same sheet music, the same vision. They meet, they plan, they use advanced virtual software to simulate the final symphony long before the day of surgery. The orthodontist sets the stage, and the surgeon performs the grand, transformative crescendo. This constant, collaborative dialogue is the silent rhythm that guarantees the success of the entire piece.

Your Journey: The Soloist in the Spotlight

This journey asks for your patience and your heart. It's a commitment of 12 to 24 months of preparation. There will be discomfort after adjustments—the feeling of the music shifting. There will be moments of doubt as you see your bite change in unfamiliar ways.

This is your solo. Your role is to trust the process, to maintain the health of your instrument with meticulous care, and to keep your eyes on the final performance. Lean on your support system, communicate with your team, and remember that every small shift is a note falling into place for the grand finale.

Without this careful, deliberate overture, the final surgery would be a gamble. The surgeon could move the bones, but the teeth wouldn't know how to meet. The result wouldn't be stable, functional, or beautiful.

Pre-surgical orthodontics is the unsung hero of your transformation. It's the dedicated, patient, and essential groundwork that ensures when the conductor's baton finally falls, the result is not just a corrected bite, but a lifelong symphony of facial harmony.

From Plaster Dust to Digital Precision: A New Dawn in Rebuilding Faces

Imagine trying to rebuild a cathedral with nothing but a chisel, a hammer, and a hand-drawn sketch. For decades, this was the world of orthognathic surgery. Surgeons and orthodontists, true artisans of their craft, would painstakingly chip away at plaster models of a patient's jaw, their hands covered in fine white dust. They were navigating by feel and experience, performing a kind of surgical prophecy on a plaster effigy, hoping the reality in the operating room would match their vision. It was a world of immense skill, but also of inherent approximation.

Today, that dusty workshop has been transformed into a digital command center, a place of stunning clarity and collaboration that feels closer to Hollywood special effects than old-world sculpting. The transformation in correcting jaws and facial structures isn't just an upgrade; it's a complete reimagining of what's possible, trading the chisel for the light of a pixel and the guess for the certainty of a thousand data points.

This new journey begins not with gooey, gag-inducing impressions, but with a quiet and elegant dance of light. First, the orthodontist wields a slender wand, an intraoral scanner, that glides through the patient's mouth. In a matter of minutes, it captures a breathtakingly detailed 3D map of every tooth and gum—a perfect, high-definition snapshot of the patient's dental universe. This isn't just a picture; it's the result of months, sometimes years, of careful orthodontic preparation, where teeth have been patiently guided into their ideal positions, poised and ready for their new home.

Then, the patient enters the quiet hum of a Cone Beam CT scanner. For a few brief moments, a gentle arc of energy passes through them, creating not a flat, shadowy X-ray, but a complete, luminous 3D model of their skull. It's like having the architectural blueprints of their entire facial structure, revealing the hidden scaffolding of bone, the delicate pathways of nerves, and the very foundation upon which their face is built.

Here, in the heart of the digital workflow, the true magic unfolds. Specialized software becomes the ultimate matchmaker, taking the intricate detail of the teeth and seamlessly "fusing" it with the profound truth of the bone. The two distinct datasets merge, blossoming into a single, breathtakingly complete virtual replica of the patient. This isn't just a model; it's a digital twin, a perfect phantom of the patient's head, ready for its transformation.

This is where the art of surgery becomes a collaborative masterpiece. The orthodontist and the surgeon meet, not over a plaster cast, but inside this shared virtual world. In a session of Virtual Surgical Planning (VSP), they become digital sculptors. With the click of a mouse, they can rotate the skull, peer into the jaw from any conceivable angle, and even make the skin transparent to see the bone beneath. It's a virtual operating room without limits.

With digital tools of microscopic precision, the surgeon can simulate the entire operation. They perform virtual "osteotomies," rehearsing the delicate cuts that will free the jaws. There is no guesswork. They can plan the exact trajectory of each incision, ensuring vital nerves are protected and the bone is perfectly prepared. Then comes the choreography. The jaws are digitally moved, gliding through space into their ideal new position. It's an iterative dance of millimeters and degrees, as the team adjusts and refines the placement to achieve a perfect bite, flawless symmetry, and a profile that brings harmony to the entire face.

But this digital foresight goes even deeper. How will the skin, lips, and chin drape over this new foundation? Sophisticated algorithms analyze the planned bone movements and generate a stunningly accurate prediction of the final facial appearance. The patient can see their future self, a powerful moment that transforms clinical anxiety into shared excitement and builds a profound bridge of trust between them and the medical team.

Once this perfect digital future is locked in, it needs a guide to bring it into the physical world. The plan is used to digitally design a surgical splint—a small, intricate guide that will nestle between the patient's teeth during the actual surgery. It is the physical key that unlocks the digital plan. This design is then beamed to a 3D printer, which, with mesmerizing precision, builds the splint layer by layer from a biocompatible resin.

When the day of surgery arrives, the surgeon walks into the operating room not with a hand-drawn map, but with a crystal-clear, scientifically validated flight plan. The 3D-printed splint acts as a perfect, unyielding guide, ensuring the jaws are moved to the exact location planned in the virtual world, down to a fraction of a millimeter. The result is a surgery that is not only dramatically more accurate and predictable but often significantly shorter, leading to quicker recoveries and profoundly better outcomes.

The revolution is in the synergy. It's in the shared vision between the orthodontist and surgeon, who now speak the same universal, visual language. It's in the empowerment of the patient, who is no longer a passive subject but an active participant in their own transformation.

We are only at the beginning of this new chapter. Soon, augmented reality may overlay the digital plan directly onto the surgeon's view in the operating room, and artificial intelligence could help design personalized solutions that are as unique as a fingerprint.

The shift from plaster to pixels is more than a technological leap; it is a changed one. It has transformed the art of rebuilding a face into a predictive science, ensuring that every patient's journey toward a new smile and a new sense of self is guided by the clearest, most precise, and most collaborative vision humanity has ever known.

The Second Sunrise: Crafting a Smile After the Storm

The day of jaw surgery feels like a mountain peak. It's the event horizon, the massive hurdle you train for, plan for, and finally, conquer. But what many don't realize is that reaching the summit is not the end of the climb. The journey that follows—the quiet, meticulous path of post-surgical orthodontics—is where the raw, powerful change from surgery is coaxed into a living, breathing masterpiece. This is not just recovery; it's a renaissance.

Waking in a New World: The First Steps

In the first weeks after surgery, you meet a stranger in the mirror. Swelling masks the new lines of your face, and your jaws, gently guided by elastics, feel both foreign and fragile. This is a sacred time of mending. The surgeon has acted as the bold architect, rebuilding the very foundation of your smile. Now, as the healing progresses, the artisan—your orthodontist—steps in to begin the intricate interior design.

When you return to the orthodontist's chair, it's a different kind of appointment. The heavy lifting is done. The goal is no longer about shifting bone, but about whispering to each tooth, guiding it home within its new, spacious architecture.

The Great Settling: Finding a Natural Harmony

Imagine building a beautiful new house. Once the walls are up and the roof is on, the house needs to settle. It needs to learn to bear its own weight, to breathe with the seasons. Your new bite is no different. The surgery set the stage, but now your body must learn the new script.

This is the "settling" phase, and it's a quiet dance between nature and science. The powerful muscles of your jaw, the gentle pressure of your tongue, the soft curtain of your lips—all are now exploring this new landscape. They are partners in the process. Your orthodontist doesn't fight these forces; they harmonize with them. With the lightest of wires and the most delicate adjustments, they encourage your teeth to find their perfect resting place, like puzzle pieces clicking satisfyingly into their final, pre-destined spots. It's a period of adaptation, where your body's own wisdom helps to perfect the surgeon's work.

The Finishing Touch: The Art of the Imperceptible

If surgery was the bold stroke of a chisel on marble, the finishing phase is the patient polishing that brings forth a human warmth and life. This is where your orthodontist's artistry shines brightest. The movements are now microscopic, often invisible to the naked eye, yet they are the difference between a good result and a breathtaking one.

This is the art of "detailing," and it's about creating a functional paradise in your mouth:

A Perfect Embrace: Each peak of a lower tooth will be guided to nestle perfectly into the valley of an upper tooth. This isn't just for looks; it's for a lifetime of comfortable chewing and shared laughter, distributing pressure so no single tooth bears too great a burden.

Aligned from the Roots Up: Below the gumline, invisible to the world, the roots of your teeth are gently encouraged to stand parallel, like strong pillars supporting a grand cathedral. This hidden alignment is the secret to a smile that will stand the test of time.

A Seamless Horizon: The edges of your teeth are smoothed into a single, flowing line, creating a smile that is not just straight, but harmonious and complete.

This stage requires patience. It can feel like watching a master painter apply single-bristle brushstrokes. But these tiny nudges are the very essence of perfection, ensuring your new smile is not just beautiful, but stable, healthy, and profoundly yours.

The Unveiling, and the Vow of a Lifetime

Then comes the day. The day the braces come off. It is a true unveiling, a moment of rediscovery. You run your tongue over smooth, unbound teeth for the first time in years. You smile at your reflection, and this time, there is no stranger—only you, reborn.

But this masterpiece is alive. And to protect it, you must make a promise. This is the beginning of retention, the most crucial act of self-custodianship. Given the monumental changes your body has accepted, the forces of memory are strong. Relapse is a shadow that lurks, and retainers are the light that keeps it at bay.

Think of your retainers not as an appliance, but as a guardian.

The fixed retainer, a discreet wire bonded behind your front teeth, is the silent, sleepless sentinel, forever standing guard over your most visible teeth.

The removable retainer, worn faithfully each night, is like a gentle embrace, holding your entire smile in a state of perfect harmony while you sleep.

Wearing them is not a chore; it's a vow. It is the lifelong commitment you make to the incredible journey you have completed, ensuring the brilliant sunrise of your new smile lasts for all your days to come.
From start to finish, this transformation is the work of a two-hearted artist: the surgeon who bravely reshaped the canvas, and the orthodontist who painstakingly perfected every detail. Together, they don't just straighten teeth or align jaws. They give you back a piece of yourself, allowing you to face the world with a confidence that is bone-deep and a smile that is, finally and forever, home.

About Author

Azhar ul Haque Sario is a bestselling author and data scientist with a remarkable record of achievement. This Cambridge alumnus brings a wealth of knowledge to his work, holding an MBA, ACCA (Knowledge Level - FTMS College Malaysia and London College of Accountancy, London), BBA, and several Google certifications, including specializations in Google Data Analytics, Google Digital Marketing & E-commerce, and Google Project Management.

With ten years of business experience, Azhar combines practical expertise with his impressive academic background to craft insightful books. His prolific writing has resulted in an astounding 2810 published titles, earning him the record for the maximum Kindle editions and paperback books published by an individual author in one year, awarded by Asia Books of Records in 2024.

ORCID: https://orcid.org/0009-0004-8629-830X
Azhar.sario@hotmail.co.uk
https://www.linkedin.com/in/azharulhaquesario/

www.ingramcontent.com/pod-product-compliance
Lightning Source LLC
Chambersburg PA
CBHW031343230926
51848CB00002B/361
9783384652980